Management of Restless Legs Syndrome

First Edition

Wayne A. Hening, MD
Assistant Clinical Professor of Neurology
UMDNJ-RW Johnson Medical School

Mark J. Buchfuhrer, MD
Medical Director, SomnoMedix Sleep Disorders
Clinic, Lakewood, CA;
Staff, Downey Regional Medical Center,
Downey, CA

Hochang B. Lee, MD
Assistant Professor of Psychiatry
and Behavioral Sciences
Johns Hopkins University School of Medicine

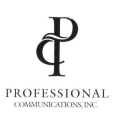

PROFESSIONAL
COMMUNICATIONS, INC.

Professional Communications, Inc.

A Medical Publishing Company

400 Center Bay Drive	PO Box 10
West Islip, NY 11795	Caddo, OK 74729-0010
(t) 631/661-2852	(t) 580/367-9838
(f) 631/661-2167	(f) 580/367-9989

For orders only, please call
1-800-337-9838
or visit our website at
www.pcibooks.com

ISBN: 978-1-932610-31-4

Printed in the United States of America

DISCLAIMER

The opinions expressed in this publication reflect those of the authors. However, the authors make no warranty regarding the contents of the publication. The protocols described herein are general and may not apply to a specific patient. Any product mentioned in this publication should be taken in accordance with the prescribing information provided by the manufacturer.

This text is printed on recycled paper.

DEDICATION

To Lucien Coté, whose wide-ranging clinical interest in unusual movement disorder patients first interested me in the study of RLS, and to Richard P. Allen, Sudhansu Chokroverty, and Christopher J. Earley who have been valuable colleagues and who have made major contributions to understanding the science and advancing the clinical management of RLS.

TABLE OF CONTENTS

TABLES

FIGURES

1
What Is RLS?

RLS is a Sensorimotor Disorder

The restless legs syndrome (RLS), named by Karl Ekbom,[1] has a name that suggests some minor irritation and, for some who have a mild case, that is all it is. But the name is misleading when applied to those who have a more severe condition, for those patients experience an almost overwhelming need to move and a discomfort that can be so excruciating it can be called "torture" (as Thomas Willis suggested about a possible case in the 17th century[2]). It also minimizes the scope of the disorder, for severe patients can have arm involvement as well and sometimes discomfort in the trunk, pelvis, and perhaps even in the face.

It is a sensorimotor disorder because it has both sensory and motor components. The sensory features are unpleasant, uncomfortable, sometimes painful feelings that can be localized to the legs (**Table 1.1**) or other affected body parts. In addition, such patients experience akathisia, a localized sense that they need to move and an inability to tolerate rest. The motor components are both voluntary and involuntary. The voluntary part is the response of the patients to their need to move—there is no specific form to this movement, although walking is the most common, but patients may stretch, bend, kick, or bicycle in order to obtain relief. They select the movement that most effectively relieves their discomfort. The involuntary part is the presence of repetitive movements that patients cannot control, periodic limb movements (PLM). These most often are present in sleep (PLM in sleep or PLMS [**Table 1.2**]) but can also occur when one is awake. For

TABLE 1.1 — Terms Used by Patients to Describe Their RLS Symptoms

- Creepy, crawly
- Insects crawling or worms wiggling in legs
- Itchy bones
- Soda in veins
- Achy pain
- Heebie-jeebies
- The "got to moves"
- The fidgets
- Electric shock feeling
- Crampy feeling

some patients, these uncontrolled jerking movements are themselves the most distressing symptom they experience. They typically recur every 10 to 40 seconds and are sometimes associated with a surge of sensory discomfort.

Is RLS a New Disorder?

For some who are just becoming aware of RLS, it may seem like a new disorder. Indeed, until the last couple of decades, RLS remained an obscure diagnosis that was rarely taught and little studied. It seems unlikely, however, that it is a truly new disorder; we can uncover literary mentions, like that of the Greek philosopher Chrysohippus who could not remain at rest during evening discussions. Many think that Willis may have been the first to describe a case in the medical literature:

> "…whilst they would indulge sleep, in their beds, immediately follow leapings up of the Tendons, in their Arms and Legs, with Cramps, and such unquietness and flying about of their members, that the sick can no more sleep, than those on the Rack." *(translated from Latin)*[3]

TABLE 1.2 — Abbreviations Associated With RLS

PLM	Periodic Limb Movement(s)—One or more movements that meet the criteria for relatively stereotyped repetitive periodic movements (criteria including number in series, period, duration, amplitude), but not restricted to the sleep state.
PLMS	Periodic Limb Movement(s) in Sleep—One or more PLM occurring in sleep. Usually used as the plural to refer to all of such movements restricted to sleep that occur during a night's study or to the condition of having such movements, generally (eg, "The patient has PLMS").
PLMW	Periodic Limb Movement(s) in Wake—One or more PLM occurring during wake.
PLMD	Periodic Limb Movement Disorder—A medical disorder with symptoms indicative of sleep disturbance. This diagnosis requires documentation of some minimum number or frequency of PLM plus some related clinical complaint such as daytime sleepiness that cannot be accounted for by another disorder. Patients with RLS cannot have PLMD.
PLMI	Periodic Limb Movement Index—Number of PLM per hour.
PLMAI	Periodic Limb Movement Arousal Index—Number of PLMS per hour of sleep associated with an arousal on polysomnography. If enumerated, one or more such movements are PLMA and their sum can be abbreviated as #PLMA.

The rack, of course, was a premodern torture device that stretched the body until it began to break. What lends greater likelihood to this description being one of RLS was Willis' treatment—laudanum, an opioid preparation that is a member of one class of drugs that have been used quite successfully to treat RLS (see Chapter 9, *Medications and Other Medical Treatments*).

The first truly comprehensive description of RLS was Ekbom's monograph[1] published in 1945, supplemented by his later papers. Ekbom appreciated that RLS is provoked by rest and that patients move in many various ways to relieve their discomfort. He understood that symptoms most likely occurred at night and that sleep could be sorely disrupted. He recognized a familial tendency and such causes as iron deficiency or pregnancy. He suggested that this was likely to be a common condition and that RLS could be readily diagnosed by a careful, pertinent clinical interview.

RLS Is a Common Condition

Ekbom found that 5% of his clinic patients could be diagnosed with RLS. While Ekbom described the symptoms of RLS, a consensus clinical definition was first promulgated by the International RLS Study Group in 1995.[4] This consensus of four clinical features (see Chapter 2, *Diagnosis and Differential Diagnosis*) led to more reliable epidemiologic studies, which confirmed that RLS is common—somewhere between 5% and 10% of adults in the community indicate that they experience these four features.[5,6] Most of the large scale studies that have used the current clinical definition have been conducted in Europe and North America. The frequency of RLS is less certain in other regions, such as Asia, but does appear to occur to some degree in all populations studied.

It is also important to define a group of those with RLS symptoms who are disturbed by the condition and merit medical attention. The REST studies delineated such a group by combining frequency of symptoms with a measure of impact: the degree to which individuals were bothered by the symptoms.[6] Those who had symptoms at least twice a week and were bothered at least moderately by symptoms when they occurred were designated as RLS sufferers. They were estimated to make up approximately 2.7% of the adult population. A recent study using actual physician diagnoses has confirmed that 2% to 3% of the adult population does suffer from RLS (*Richard Allen, personal communication, June 2007*). While less common in children, such clinically significant RLS is not rare; about 1% of teenagers are RLS sufferers and even ½% of younger children.[7] These numbers are such that every physician will come into contact with patients who have RLS that merits intervention; some physicians—particularly those in specialties dealing with secondary RLS (due to pregnancy, iron deficiency, kidney failure, neuropathy, diabetes, rheumatoid arthritis)—are likely to see many such patients.

RLS Causes Significant Morbidity

The symptoms of RLS are themselves bothersome; patients dislike having them and strive to avoid them. But this often requires avoiding personally meaningful activities that might provoke symptoms: lectures, conferences, desk work, theater, travel, dinner parties, and so on. Some patients cannot sit and watch TV or even sit and work on a computer. Virginia Wilson, a patient advocate who brought into being the first book on RLS for the general public,[8] had to prepare her manuscript while standing up, continually moving her feet to avoid her RLS. Other patients have had to quit their chosen occupations: Ekbom, for instance, mentions a truck driver who had symptoms whenever driving and had to abandon that line of work.

A major problem in RLS patients and the complaint that historically has most led patients to seek medical attention for their symptoms is the disruption of sleep. Because of their symptoms, they may find it difficult to get to sleep. When they awaken, perhaps caused by PLMS, they may have a reactivation of their symptoms. Patients with severe PLMS may experience only a few hours of fragmented sleep in the course of the night—a degree of sleep deprivation equal to, if not exceeding, that of any other sleep disorder.[9]

Their sleep problems then become the basis for further morbidities.[10] These problems include fatigue, difficulty concentrating, depressed mood, and excessive daytime sleepiness. Thinking and judgment can be impaired. Studies have now shown that RLS patients are more likely to have anxiety disorders and depression, even compared with those with other chronic disorders.[11] The RLS patients were also more likely to attribute their mood disorders to their symptoms than were the controls. Recent studies have even suggested that RLS may be associated with physical disorders, such as hypertension and cardiovascular disease.[12] While these cross-sectional studies do not establish RLS as the cause of the psychiatric and medical disorders, they do raise the possibility and underline the importance of the condition.

In summary, RLS is not a trivial disease. While those with rarely occurring symptoms can easily adapt to their condition, the 2% to 3% of adults with significant disease represent an important clinical challenge. It is clearly not "disease mongering" to recommend the appropriate diagnosis and treatment of such patients—a population that too often went without diagnosis or appropriate treatment in the past.[13] To vividly illustrate the historical frustration and lack of treatment of these patients, it is instructive to read the many personal testimonials in a recent book by Robert Yoakum, another

RLS sufferer.[14] For many patients with severe RLS, it is the worst problem of their lives.

The aim of this book is to provide the tools necessary to accurately diagnose and appropriately treat RLS patients. The bulk of the text will be devoted to this aim. For background, we will provide some information about the epidemiology, genetics, and pathophysiology of the condition. We will also provide information about the range of RLS patients—both idiopathic and secondary—that may be encountered in different practices and the special requirements for their treatment. Our emphasis will be on the basics of managing RLS, but we will include enough information to facilitate the management of the more difficult or complicated patient.

REFERENCES

1. Ekbom KA. Restless legs: a clinical study. *Acta Med Scand Supplementum.* 1945;158(suppl):1-122.
2. Willis T. *De Animae Brutorum.* London: Wells and Scott; 1672.
3. Willis T. *Two Discourses Concerning the Soul of Brutes.* London: Dring, Harper, and Leigh; 1683.
4. Walters AS. Toward a better definition of the restless legs syndrome. The International Restless Legs Syndrome Study Group. *Mov Disord.* 1995;10(5):634-642.
5. Berger K, Luedemann J, Trenkwalder C, John U, Kessler C. Sex and the risk of restless legs syndrome in the general population. *Arch Intern Med.* 2004;164(2):196-202.
6. Allen RP, Walters AS, Montplaisir J, et al. Restless legs syndrome prevalence and impact: REST general population study. *Arch Intern Med.* 2005;165(11):1286-1292.
7. Picchietti D, Allen RP, Walters AS, Davidson JE, Myers A, Ferini-Strambi L. Restless legs syndrome: prevalence and impact in children and adolescents—the Peds REST study. *Pediatrics.* 2007;120(2):253-266.
8. Wilson VN, Buchholz D, Walters AS. *Sleep Thief: Restless Legs Syndrome.* Orange Park, FL: Galaxy Books; 1996.
9. Allen RP, Earley CJ. Restless legs syndrome: a review of clinical and pathophysiologic features. *J Clin Neurophysiol.* 2001;18(2):128-147.

10. Kushida CA, Allen RP, Atkinson MJ. Modeling the causal relationships between symptoms associated with restless legs syndrome and the patient-reported impact of RLS. *Sleep Med.* 2004;5(5):485-488.

11. Winkelmann J, Prager M, Lieb R, et al. "Anxietas tibiarum." Depression and anxiety disorders in patients with restless legs syndrome. *J Neurol.* 2005;252(1):67-71.

12. Winkelman JW, Finn L, Young T. Prevalence and correlates of restless legs syndrome symptoms in the Wisconsin Sleep Cohort. *Sleep Med.* 2006;7(7):545-552.

13. Hening W, Walters AS, Allen RP, Montplaisir J, Myers A, Ferini-Strambi L. Impact, diagnosis and treatment of restless legs syndrome (RLS) in a primary care population: the REST (RLS epidemiology, symptoms, and treatment) primary care study. *Sleep Med.* 2004;5(3):237-246.

14. Yoakum R. *Restless Legs Syndrome: Relief and Hope for Sleepless Victims of a Hidden Epidemic.* New York: Fireside; 2006.

2

Diagnosis and Differential Diagnosis

Diagnosis of RLS

■ **The Four Diagnostic Features**: **URGE**

The diagnosis of restless legs syndrome (RLS) is a clinical diagnosis. There are no specific tests to order, no pathognomic findings on exam or in the laboratory. Diagnosis depends on the patient's history of symptoms. As developed by the International RLS Study Group,[1,2] there are four diagnostic features that must be present to make a definite diagnosis of RLS (**Table 2.1**). These can be remembered under the acronym **URGE** (**Table 2.2**). This acronym emphasizes the key symptom of RLS: an urge to move the legs, usually accompanied or caused by unpleasant, uncomfortable sensations in the legs. The other three diagnostic features indicate those situations that provoke or ameliorate the urge (or akathisia).

Urge to Move the Legs

The urge or need to move in RLS is a specific impression that is localized to the legs. The most common expression of patients when asked about their symptoms is "I just have to move. I can't keep still." This is not some generalized anxiety or unsettled feeling, but a specific feeling in the legs: Patients can point to the location of their symptoms. The urge to move is also not an observation or judgment; the patient must experience the urge. The individuals who may frequently tap their feet or shake their legs may have RLS, but if they are unaware of their movement until their attention is called to it and cannot describe

TABLE 2.1 — The Four Diagnostic Features of RLS
1. An urge to move the legs that is usually accompanied or caused by unpleasant sensations in the legs 2. The worsening of the symptoms at rest 3. The relief of symptoms with activity 4. A variation of symptoms with time of day such that symptoms are worse or only occur in the evening and/or night
In severe cases, it may be difficult to show that there is relief with activity or a worsening later in the day, because the symptoms may persist whenever the patient is awake and may require continuous activity to keep them suppressed. In such cases, the patient will generally report that the symptoms varied with time of day and were suppressed by activity earlier in the course.

TABLE 2.2 — URGE: The Four Clinical Features of RLS
• Urge to move the legs • Rest induced • Gets better with activity • Evening and night worse

an actual need to move, they do not have RLS. Most patients with severe RLS say that when they have the urge, they cannot resist moving their legs.

Most patients can also describe an unpleasant sensation in the legs, although a minority of patients deny an unpleasant sensation and only describe an isolated urge to move. Those who report sensations may attribute their need to move to this symptom, which may be described in a very wide variety of ways (**Table 1.1**). Almost invariably, the sensation will be described using negative terms. Typically, the sensation is experienced within the limb, in the muscles, or in bones. It is less likely to be felt in the joints or in the feet, although such a distribution does occur. The most common location is between knee and ankle, although symptoms frequently occur above the knee. In most patients, the feeling is bilateral, although often one leg is more involved than the other. Rarely, the feeling may be unilateral. The site and the laterality of the symptoms may vary from night to night; a few patients report that their legs alternate with only a single leg symptomatic on a given night. It is uncommon for the feeling to be localized to the skin surface. The area of involvement is usually nontender; rubbing or massaging the skin over the sensation tends to bring relief rather than provoking additional discomfort

The primary symptom of RLS is a persistent feeling that will last for a sustained period until the patient moves. It is not a brief or fleeting feeling and it is not specifically positional. It is only briefly or occasionally relieved by a change of posture; sustained relief requires actual continuous movement. Some patients may say that their symptoms are brief, but if asked the period of time before they can have relief without movement, they indicate that this is many minutes or even hours before symptoms no longer persist.

Patients with severe RLS frequently experience their RLS symptoms outside of the legs. Most commonly, symptoms are felt in the arms.[3] Less commonly, the hips, trunk, shoulders, genitals, or anal region may be involved. The patient will describe the sensation in the extended area as being the same or very similar to that in the legs and it will be generally modulated by the same factors (features 2 to 4). Typically, arm symptoms are experienced less frequently than those in the legs and begin later in the course of the disorder. It is distinctly unusual for the arm symptoms or symptoms in other regions to develop prior to leg symptoms or to be the sole or major manifestation of the condition.

The majority of those with RLS symptoms differentiate their symptoms from pain; the symptoms are definitely unpleasant, but not painful. However, pain is a common descriptor for those with more frequent and severe symptoms, reaching the majority in at least one case series.[4] In our experience, almost all patients who say their symptoms are painful liken them to an ache. Almost all of them will judge that a muscle cramp, which occurs on some occasion to almost all individuals, provides a pain of a different order and intensity—a sharp, severe pain as opposed to the ache of RLS symptoms.

Rest Induced

RLS symptoms are evoked by rest. Patients are readily aware that if they sit or lie down, they will develop symptoms after a period of time. The rapidity of symptom onset is one measure of the severity of RLS symptoms. If symptoms begin while a patient is active, this is very unlikely to be caused by RLS. However, patients with severe RLS may experience symptoms while standing quietly and symptoms may persist as they begin to move around.

Rest is a general state; it implies both lack of motor activity and a general easing of alertness. It should not be position dependent. For most patients, lying is more likely to produce symptoms than sitting upright. In the Johns Hopkins family study, a diagnosis of definite RLS required that the person have more than rare symptoms when lying down.[5] There does seem, however, to be a group of younger individuals who experience RLS only when sitting; they can easily get to sleep before they have been lying long enough to develop any symptoms. Such individuals usually have relatively mild RLS. A more persistent state of rest (eg, during theater, dinner parties, travel) can cause symptoms even in the daytime, when they are generally uncommon.

Particularly difficult for RLS patients is a state of confinement. An airplane flight is a classic example of confinement, especially in a seat with restricted room and blocked access to the aisle. RLS patients generally indicate that they would be very troubled by a situation in which they were unable to freely move. This could lead to great mental stress, panic, and whatever movement is possible in the situation. Studies have shown that, when patients are required to remain at rest, symptoms will increase at least in the first hour at any time of day.[6,7]

Relieved by Movement

Patients with RLS readily discover that movement can relieve their symptoms. This relief generally lasts as long as the movement continues. The most typical movement is walking, but various movements while in place can occur, such as flexing and extending the legs, stretching the legs, pumping the legs, shaking the legs, or moving the trunk or arms; these may all relieve leg discomfort. Relief generally begins quickly; many patients report that they begin to feel better almost immediately when they have begun to move. For some patients, however, it takes more time for relief. This is particularly true of patients with very severe RLS. Elderly patients with compromised mobility may find that it is difficult for them to achieve a level of movement that is adequate to provide complete relief.

Two other forms of activity provide relief. One is mental—an exciting or stimulating activity that may not require much actual movement, such as game playing, watching a stimulating movie, or even arguing, can provide relief. The other is sensory; patients may report that massage, striking the leg, applying pressure, or rubbing on lotion may provide relief. In some, sexual activity can also provide at least temporary relief.

If asked, patients with severe RLS may report that they do not obtain relief with movement, but often they mean that movement does not provide continuing relief: once they sit or lie back down, they find that the discomfort quickly returns. However, during the period of movement, they do obtain relief. In a patient who can walk normally, relief should persist as long as the movement continues. Moreover, RLS symptoms should never begin during active movement.

Evening or Night Worse

Most patients indicate that their symptoms are worse at night or only occur at night. The exceptions are those patients so severe that they can have symptoms at any time with sufficient rest or those who are so mild that they only experience symptoms when, while awake, they must remain at rest for a prolonged period. However, the time period that is most severe can vary between patients from the evening (in patients who may be able to get to sleep quickly before their symptoms are provoked), to bedtime to later in the night. While some patients only have symptoms in one of these periods, patients with more severe RLS may have symptoms that begin in the evening or even earlier in the day and persist through much of the night. They may have difficulty falling asleep and staying asleep because of their symptoms.

Initially, it was thought that symptoms were only worse in the evening because that was when rest occurred; in other words, that this fourth criterion was only a corollary of the second (rest induced). However, several studies have now established that the symptoms of RLS follow a true circadian pattern, with severity maximal during the early part of the night (23:00 to 4:00) and a protected period early in the day (9:00 to 13:00).[8,9] By having patients follow a constant routine and requiring multiple periods of rest (using a suggested immobilization test [**Table 2**.3]), it was possible to show that the circadian alteration of symptoms was not caused by rest alone, but also depended on time of day. It also did not depend on period of sleep deprivation since symptoms were also reduced during

TABLE 2.3 — Procedure for Suggested Immobilization Test

- Subject sits with legs outstretched, usually on a bed
- Subject is instructed not to move unless it is absolutely necessary
- No diverting activity is permitted (no television, reading, radio, talking)
- One or more leg symptoms are monitored by questionnaire or visual analogue scale (VAS) at intervals of 5 to 15 minutes
- Leg movements (or activity) are measured by electromyelogram (EMG) on the tibialis anterior or actigraphy of the legs
- The subject is monitored visually or by sleep recording to ensure that sleep does not occur

the protected period after a night of sleep deprivation. Symptoms occurred during the falling phase of core body temperature and began to improve as core temperature rose in the period before waking (**Figure 2.1**).[8,9] One study measured another circadian marker, melatonin, which begins to rise within a few hours of normal bedtime and remains elevated during the night, decreasing as the sleep period ends.[10] In that study, it could be seen that the RLS symptoms were maximal during the period when melatonin was elevated. The relationship of RLS symptoms to the overall circadian rhythm controlled by the suprachiasmatic nucleus is unclear. Although one group has suggested that melatonin, which suppresses dopamine, may be partly responsible for the nocturnal peak of RLS symptoms,[10] this link remains to be proven. One manifestation of the circadian accentuation of RLS is the more rapid development of RLS symptoms during the late evening and night.[6,7]

One finding of these circadian studies is that at least in severe RLS patients, symptoms can be provoked at any time of day with sufficient imposed rest.[7-9]

FIGURE 2.1 — Circadian Rhythm of RLS and Core Temperature

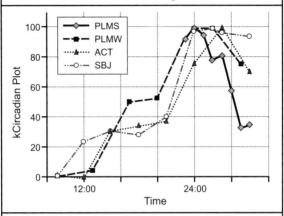

Abbreviations: ACT, activity accounts (measure of motor restlessness); mSIT, modified SIT to allow restless movement to alleviate symptoms; PLMS, periodic limb movements in sleep; PSG, polysomnography; PLMW, periodic limb movements while awake; SBJ, subjective leg discomfort; SIT, suggested immobilization test.

Circadian composite figure (reporting data from two studies[1,2]). Normalized values of the RLS measures are plotted against clock time from 8:00 through 24:00 to 8:00. Hours represent beginning of a SIT period or beginning of an hour of enumerating PLMS. Hourly averages from the first study from 23:00 to 7:00 are plotted as percent of the maximum (94.9 per hour in the period from 24:00 to 1:00). Mean value for eight subjects and two nights PSG. All these are plotted as percent from minimum (0%) to maximum (100%). PLMW[1]—minimum of 13.8/hour (9:00), maximum of 91.5/hour (2:00). ACT[2]—minimum of 124.9 counts (12:00), maximum of 447.8 (3:00). SBJ[2]—minimum of 2.96 (on 0 to 10 scale averaged over 5 determinations per 1 hour mSIT) at 9:00; maximum of 6.04 (at 12:00). The values of PLMW[1], ACT[2], and SBJ[2] were taken by averaging daytime SITs (or mSITs) from the first 2 days of study; values from hours between 11:00 and 6:00 were taken from the night of sleep deprivation.

[1]Trenkwalder C, et al. *Mov Disord.* 1999;14:102-110; [2]Hening WA, et al. *Sleep.* 1999;22:901-912.

This possibility can become important when patients develop augmentation (see Chapter 9, *Medications and Other Medical Treatments*). It may also have clinical relevance when the alleviation of nighttime symptoms leads to a greater salience of afternoon ones. Therefore, even without the advance to early hours of augmentation, treated patients may begin to feel that they need relief earlier in the day.

Differential Diagnosis of RLS: Discrimination from Mimics

■ The Mimics of RLS

There are two main categories of conditions that can be confused with RLS. First, there is the condition of restlessness, which can range from true akathisia to generalized anxiety. These have some relation to RLS since the most severe or augmented RLS can resemble generalized akathisia and the symptoms of anxiety are both common in RLS and partially overlap the key features of RLS.[11] The main overlap is in an urge to move or discomfort at rest. **Table 2.4** lists the disorders in this category. Second, there are those disorders that involve pain or unpleasant feelings in the legs. Leg cramps, known in the United States as "charley horses," are typical of this category. **Table 2.5** lists disorders in this category of leg discomfort.

It should be remembered, however, that RLS can be comorbid with some of the conditions that are in the differential diagnosis, such as rheumatoid arthritis,[12] diabetic neuropathy,[13] or other pain syndromes.[14] These situations in which symptoms overlap can present some of the most difficult diagnostic issues.

How to Avoid Misdiagnosis

The first step in the differential diagnosis of RLS is to probe for the presence of the four diagnostic features. For a secure diagnosis, all four must be present. Many

TABLE 2.4 — Disorders of Restlessness

Akathisia
- Due to neuroleptic or other dopamine-blocking medications
- Due to other classes of psychoactive compounds, such as selective serotonin reuptake inhibitors (SSRIs)
- Due to degenerative disease
- Idiopathic

Anxiety Disorders

Other Psychiatric Disorders
- Mania
- Obsessive-compulsive disorder

Repetitive Movement Habits
- Leg shaking
- Foot tapping

Leg Symptoms With Toe Dyskinesias
- Painful legs and moving toes
- "Painless legs" and moving toes

Movement Disorders[1]
- Hypnic jerks
- Propriospinal myoclonus at sleep onset
- Tic disorder
- Hypnic myoclonus:
  – Excessive fragmentary myoclonus
- Rhythmic movement disorder:
  – Hypnic foot tremor
  – Alternating leg movement activity

[1] American Sleep Disorders Association. *The International Classification of Sleep Disorders: Diagnostic and Coding Manual*, 2nd Version. Chicago, IL: American Association of Sleep Disorders; 2005.

of the mimic conditions will fail one or more of the four diagnostic features, such as the presence of an experienced urge to move or the lack of any history of a nighttime accentuation. In addition, some mimics that might cause problems for an epidemiologic study, such as positional discomfort or occasional nocturnal leg cramps, are unlikely to present within a clinical practice.

TABLE 2.5 — Disorders of Leg Discomfort
Cramps   • Nocturnal leg cramps   • Metabolic cramps   • Myopathic cramps
Arthritic Conditions   • Rheumatoid arthritis   • Osteoarthritis
Pain Syndromes   • Fibromyalgia   • Somatiform pain disorder
Vascular Disorders   • Claudication   • Varicose veins   • Berger's disease   • Diabetic small-vessel disease

Nerve Disorders
 • Polyneuropathies:
    – Small-fiber neuropathies
    – Diabetic neuropathy
 • Radiculopathies

The next step, in doubtful cases, is to probe more deeply into the nature of the four features; some helpful questions to ask are given in **Table 2.6**. Such questioning may be necessary because simply asking about the four diagnostic features may not fully establish the core elements of the features.

In addition, there are aspects of RLS symptoms that go beyond the four features. You can ask about specific ways in which the symptoms manifest. A list of potential questions with an explanation of how the answers influence diagnosis is presented in **Table 2.7**.

Finally, there are features of patient presentation in history or on exam that can be used to discriminate different mimic conditions from RLS. Some of these are presented in **Table 2.8**. In cases with atypical features, such as arm predominance or the lack of any symptoms when at rest, one of the supportive features

TABLE 2.6 — Additional Questions to Ask to Elucidate the Four Diagnostic Features of RLS

Urge to Move
- Do you experience this urge within your legs?
- Is the need to move overwhelming to the point that you cannot resist moving your legs?
- Will the urge to move increase if you are in a confined position?

Provocation by Rest
- Do you have symptoms both sitting and lying?
- How long do you need to be at rest before your leg symptoms begin?
- Do your symptoms only begin when your legs are in a specific posture?

Relief by Activity
- How quickly do you get some relief when you start moving?
- Do your leg symptoms ever occur when you are walking?
- Do your leg symptoms ever start when you are walking?
- If you have obtained relief with walking, do the symptoms ever return while you continue to walk?

Circadian Rhythm
- When are your symptoms worst?
- When are your symptoms least?
- Do you find that your symptoms are less in the morning?

may help clarify the diagnosis or at least direct further investigation.

Supportive RLS Diagnostic Features

The 2002 IRLSSG-NIH consensus conference on RLS diagnosis indicated three specific findings that might enhance the likelihood of RLS diagnosis (**Table 2.9**); these include:
- The presence of periodic limb movements (PLM)
- The response of symptoms to dopaminergics
- A positive family history.

**TABLE 2.7 — Other Questions to
Differentiate RLS From Mimics**

1. How long do your symptoms last until you have full relief (you no longer need to move to obtain relief)?
   Restless leg syndrome (RLS) symptoms usually last at least 10 minutes and often hours before full relief is obtained.

2. Are your symptoms relieved if you merely make a single change in the posture of your legs?
   RLS symptoms are only briefly or occasionally benefited by a postural shift; in general, one shift will not have more than a transitory effect on a state of rest.

3. Are your symptoms like a sharp pain?
   While RLS symptoms may be described as painful, they generally present as a diffuse pain or ache.

4. Does pressing the involved part of the leg cause additional pain?
   In RLS, there is normally not tenderness; instead, pressing or rubbing may relieve discomfort.

■ **Periodic Limb Movements**

These are repetitive leg movements that are most likely to occur during sleep, but especially in RLS also occur while awake. Their tight association with RLS was first determined by the Lugaresi group in Bologna in the mid 1960s.[15,16] Recently, their identification was operationalized,[17] as reflected in the new International Classification of Sleep Disorders-2[18] and the new American Sleep Scoring Manual.[19] The criteria for PLM are given in **Table 2.10**. These movements occur in series of four or more (by definition) and typically recur at intervals of 10 to 50 seconds (**Figure 2.2**) that can vary in period and amplitude with sleep/wake states.[20] As shown in the figure, the arms as well as the legs may be involved in the periodic limb movements in sleep (PLMS).[21] Most PLMS (see **Table 1.2** for definitions) occur during stages 1 and 2 non–rapid eye movement (NREM) sleep. Periodic

TABLE 2.8 — Specific Issues in Differential Diagnosis

Disorder	Key Point
Akathisia	Can usually identify the causative agent
Anxiety	Even if there is a circadian rhythm, specific symptoms in the legs are absent
Leg shaking/foot tapping	Usually do not experience an urge to move
Painful legs and moving toes	Exam discloses 1 to 2 Hz movements of the toes
Cramps	Usually intensely painful with obvious muscle contraction
Arthritis	Location of pain and signs to the joints
Pain syndromes	May have no urge to move and unusual distribution
Nerve disorders	Frequent numbness and signs of muscle wasting

TABLE 2.9 — Supportive Criteria for the Diagnosis of RLS

- The presence of an increased number or frequency of periodic limb movements for age
- The relief of symptoms by dopaminergic medications
- A family history of restless legs syndrome in close family members

Modified from: Allen RP, et al. *Sleep Med.* 2003;4(2):101-119.

TABLE 2.10 — Current Diagnosis of Periodic Limb Movement

- Each movement (measured by electromyelogram [EMG] or actigraphy) lasts between 0.5 and 10 seconds
- The period of movements (interval from onset to onset) is at least 5 and not >90 seconds.
- For EMG, movement is said to begin when the rectified EMG rises 8 microvolts above baseline
- For EMG, movement is said to end when the rectified EMG falls below 2 microvolts above baseline for 0.5 seconds
- Movements must be separated by at least 0.5 seconds
- If a movement in one leg begins within 5 seconds of a movement in the other, it can be considered as part of the same movement
- At least four consecutive movements must meet the above criteria

Adapted from: Zucconi M, et al. *Sleep Med.* 2006;7(2):175-183.

increases and amplitude decreases in slower NREM sleep.[22] In REM sleep, amplitude and period may both decrease. In wake, periodic limb movements in wake (PLMW) may be more irregular with a shorter period and a more prolonged duration of muscular activity that often includes muscular jerks.[23] These prolonged movements may include voluntary components evoked by the involuntary PLMW. One recent effort has been to impose a specific criterion of periodicity on these

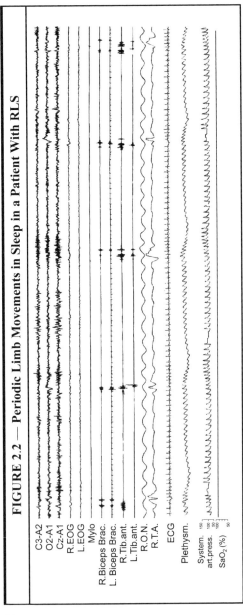

FIGURE 2.2 — Periodic Limb Movements in Sleep in a Patient With RLS

Abbreviations: Biceps Brac, biceps brachii; ECG, electrocardiogram; EOG, electrooculogram; L, left; Mylo, mylohyoideus; Plethysm, plethysmogram; PLMS, periodic limb movements during sleep; R, right; RON, oronasal respirogram; RTA, thoracoabdominal respirogram; SaO$_2$, oxygen saturation; System art press, Systemic arterial pressure; Tib. ant., Tibialis anterior.

Contractions synchronously involve lower- and upper-limb muscles, recurring periodically about every 20 seconds. Note the ECG (heart rate) and plethysmogram (blood pressure) increases associated with the PLMS.

Courtesy of the Bologna Sleep Neurology group, Drs. Provini, Vertrugno, and Montagna.

movements: How regular are the successive intervals between movements.[24] In RLS, compared with other conditions, the PLMS are more regular, more strictly periodic. This is reflected in an index that forms a ratio between more periodic and less periodic movements.

Epidemiology of PLM

PLM are by no means restricted to RLS, although there seems to be an important pathophysiologic connection between RLS as reflected in the association of PLMS with RLS in two reported genetic linkages, 12q[25] and 14q,[26,27] as well as one of the genes associated with RLS, BTB09 (6p).[27] One recent study also suggested that the rise of PLMS in older individuals may be accentuated in those who are related to individuals with RLS,[28] consistent with genetic determinants that are common to RLS and increased PLM.

Most studies of PLM have focused on those that occur during sleep or PLMS (see **Table 1.2** for definitions). It was early noted that there are frequent PLMS in the elderly.[29,30] More recent studies in a general population indicate that PLMS are relatively infrequent (<5/hour of sleep) in early decades, but increase rapidly after age 40 and may continue to increase in older age groups (**Figure 2.3**).[31] In addition, PLMS in older subjects tend to be more rhythmic.

Table 2.11 lists conditions in which frequent PLMS have been found. Particularly noteworthy are such sleep neurologic conditions such as narcolepsy[32,33] and REM sleep behavior disorder,[34,35] two conditions that may also co-occur.[34]

Association of PLM With RLS and Diagnostic Utility

The difficulty with using PLM as a diagnostic measure of RLS is that PLM are not specific for RLS. The Montreal group under Jacques Montplaisir has most investigated the diagnostic utility of PLM for

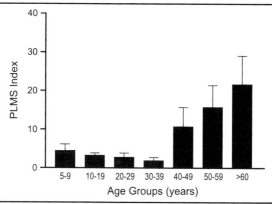

FIGURE 2.3 — Distribution of Periodic Limb Movements During Sleep by Age

Mean periodic limb movements during sleep (PLMS) index for healthy subjects according to 7 age groups (5-9 y, 10-19 y, 20-29 y, 30-39 y, 40-49 y, 50-59 y, and 60 y and older). Vertical bars represent the SEM.

Pennestri MH, et al. *Sleep*. 2006;29:1183-1187.

TABLE 2.11 — Conditions Other Than RLS With Frequent Periodic Limb Movement In Sleep

- Rapid eye movement behavior disorder
- Narcolepsy
- Synucleinopathies
  - Parkinson's disease
  - Multiple-system atrophy
- Pregnancy (especially multiple pregnancies)
- Heart failure (post-transplant)
- Obstructive sleep apnea
- Antidepressant therapy
  - Selective serotonin reuptake inhibitors
  - Tricyclic agents
  - Lithium

RLS. In an early study, the group found that 80% of RLS patients have >5 PLMS/hour sleep.[36] Subsequent studies used a combination of a suggested immobilization test (SIT) with a polysomnographic (PSG) sleep study to determine how well these two studies in combination could differentiate between RLS patients and normal controls.[37] Using the measure of sensory discomfort in the SIT (subject ratings using a 10-point visual analogue scale [VAS] combined with the index of PLMW during the PSG [PLMW/hour of wake]) could best differentiate RLS patients from controls, with a sensitivity of 82% and a specificity of 100%. Therefore, the combination of high discomfort on the SIT and frequent PLMW at night is very uncommon in those who have few sleep complaints. On the other hand, the optimized measures they chose were not met by one of six RLS patients. The problem with this analysis is that it is unclear that when a more difficult differential diagnosis is required, say between RLS and polyneuropathy, a similarly effective discrimination can be made.

As discussed in the evaluation section of Chapter 3, *Who Gets RLS and How Does It Progress?*, a PSG is not indicated for routine diagnosis of RLS. However, the detection of PLMS themselves does require a PSG and can be a rationale for performing such a study. If that alternative is not available, a new technology that is available is actigraphy. Small, accelerometer-based instruments that can be worn for several days and record and count PLM can be used to measure PLM.[38] These have the advantage that they are relatively inexpensive and allow for a more sustained recording. This is useful since PLM may vary from day to day and can be better characterized with multiday recording.[39]

Periodic Limb Movement Disorder
An unresolved issue in sleep medicine is the clinical significance of PLMS.[40] Patients can have many

PLMS and no sleep complaints, even PLMS associated with arousals that are thought to impair the quality of sleep.[41] Periodic limb movement disorder (PLMD) is a diagnosis in which PLMS are found to cause a specific complaint of disrupted sleep or excessive daytime sleepiness[18]: Specific diagnostic criteria are given in **Table 2.12**.

To reach a diagnosis of PLMD, no other sleep-related diagnosis can account for the patient's complaint. It is a rule that leg movements, even if periodic, are not considered to be PLM if they are associated regularly with respiratory disturbances, such as sleep apnea.[18] A respiratory disturbance of increased pressure and turbulence, usually heard as snoring, is called upper airway resistance syndrome (UARS).[42] To discover this condition requires monitoring of nasal or esophageal pressure, which has not been standard in PSGs in the past, but is becoming more common today. It is therefore thought that many cases of insomnia or daytime sleepiness thought due to PLMD were actually caused by UARS. As a consequence of the definition of PLMD, a patient with RLS cannot have PLMD. These differences are shown in **Table 2.13**.

More recently, it has been noted that there may be an association between PLMS and autonomic activation, including increases in heart rate and blood pressure. The effect is greater if the PLMS are associated with an arousal.[43] It is speculated that this may be a risk factor for the development of cardiovascular disease, which has recently been associated with RLS.[44] If PLMS do have this effect, they will clearly be seen as more clinically important and treatment of them, which is today relatively optional, may be seen as necessary.

■ **Response to Dopaminergic Medications**

Dopaminergic medications were early discovered to benefit RLS. Beginning with Akpinar's original report of 1982,[45] the vast majority of studies with dopa-

TABLE 2.12 — Diagnostic Criteria for Periodic Limb Movement Disorder

- Polysomnography demonstrates repetitive, highly stereotyped limb movements that are:
  - 0.5 to 5 seconds in duration;
  - In a sequence of four or more movements
  - Separated by an interval of >5 seconds (from limb movement onset to limb movement onset) and <90 seconds (typically there is an interval of 20 seconds to 40 seconds)*
- The PLMS Index exceeds five per hour in children and 15 per hour in most adult cases.
- There is clinical sleep disturbance or complaints of daytime fatigue. If PLMS are present without clinical sleep disturbance, the PLMS can be noted as a polysomnographic finding, but criteria are not met for a diagnosis of PLMD.
- The periodic limb movements are not better explained by another current sleep disorder, medical/neurologic disorder, medication use, or substance use disorder. An example would be the occurrence of periodic leg movements at the termination of cyclically occurring apneas, which should not be counted as true PLMS or PLMD

Abbreviations: ICSD, International Classification iof Sleep Disorders; PLMS, periodic limb movement in sleep; PLMD, periodic limb movement disorder.

* The ICSD2 criteria use an obsolete measure of amplitude, which is no longer accepted.

Adapted from: American Sleep Disorders Association. *The International Classification of Sleep Disorders: Diagnostic and Coding Manual*, 2nd Version. Chicago, IL: American Association of Sleep Disorders; 2005.

minergics in RLS have been successful.[46,47] This led to the suggestion that a failure of a previously untreated patient to respond promptly to a dopaminergic would raise questions about an RLS diagnosis. In one study, individuals with possible RLS, not fulfilling all criteria,

2

TABLE 2.13 — Differences Between RLS and Periodic Limb Movement Disorder

	RLS	PLMD
Diagnosis	Clinical history with exclusion of mimics	Documentation of PLMS of sufficient quantity by PSG (or possibly actigraphy)
Complaint	Typical leg symptoms satisfying clinical features	Complaint of sleep disturbance or daytime excessive somnolence
Differential diagnosis	A variet of disorders involving an urge to move and leg complaints	Movement disorders of sleep, such as nocturnal epilepsy, RBD, rhythmic movement disorder
Treatment	Dopaminergics, anticonvulsants, opioids, sedative-hypnotics	Mostly dopaminergics, sedative-hypnotics, some anticonvulsants

Abbreviations: PLMD, periodic limb movement disorder; PLMS, periodic limb movement in sleep; PSG, polysomnography; RBD, REM behavior disorder.

were tested by administering a single 100-mg dose of levodopa when they were symptomatic.[48] They then completed a VAS scale for their RLS-like symptoms (urge to move and leg discomfort); those who showed a ≥50% benefit on the scale were subsequently found to have true RLS. Based on the two scales, 83% and 90% of those with true RLS were identified. This study then reinforces the clinical impression that giving a single levodopa dose in doubtful cases may assist with diagnosis. Further evaluation is required to establish more precisely how valuable such a test may be.

■ Presence of a Positive Family History

As explained in Chapter 4, *Pathophysiology*, RLS is a familial disease with likely genetic bases. Because of this, someone related to a known RLS patient is up to six times more likely to have RLS. These individuals are likely to be more familiar with the condition and better understand the symptoms. There are no studies on how useful a known positive family history is in uncertain cases, but family history is an important element of diagnosis in cases of pediatric RLS (see *Chapter 3*).

REFERENCES

1. Walters AS. Toward a better definition of the restless legs syndrome. International Restless Legs Syndrome Study Group. *Mov Disord.* 1995;10:634-642.
2. Allen RP, Picchietti D, Hening WA, et al. Restless legs syndrome: diagnostic criteria, special considerations, and epidemiology. A report from the restless legs syndrome diagnosis and epidemiology workshop at the National Institutes of Health. *Sleep Med.* 2003;4:101-119.
3. Michaud M, Chabli A, Lavigne G, Montplaisir J. Arm restlessness in patients with restless legs syndrome. *Mov Disord.* 2000;15:289-293.
4. Bassetti CL, Mauerhofer D, Gugger M, Mathis J, Hess CW. Restless legs syndrome: a clinical study of 55 patients. *Eur Neurol.* 2001;45:67-74.
5. Hening W, Washburn M, Allen R, Lesage S, Earley C. Validation of the Hopkins telephone diagnostic interview for the restless legs syndrome. *Sleep Med.* 2007 Jul 16. Epub ahead of print.
6. Michaud M, Dumont M, Paquet J, Desautels A, Fantini ML, Montplaisir J. Circadian variation of the effects of immobility on symptoms of restless legs syndrome. *Sleep.* 2005;28:843-846.
7. Allen RP, Dean T, Earley CJ. Effects of rest-duration, time-of-day and their interaction on periodic leg movements while awake in restless legs syndrome. *Sleep Med.* 2005;6:429-434.
8. Trenkwalder C, Hening WA, Walters AS, Campbell SS, Rahman K, Chokroverty S. Circadian rhythm of periodic limb movements and sensory symptoms of restless legs syndrome. *Mov Disord.* 1999;14:102-110.
9. Hening WA, Walters AS, Wagner M, et al. Circadian rhythm of motor restlessness and sensory symptoms in the idiopathic restless legs syndrome. *Sleep.* 1999;22:901-912.

10. Michaud M, Dumont M, Selmaoui B, Paquet J, Fantini ML, Montplaisir J. Circadian rhythm of restless legs syndrome: relationship with biological markers. *Ann Neurol.* 2004;55:372-380.

11. Lee HB, Hening WA, Allen RP, et al. Restless legs syndrome is associated with DSM IV major depressive disorder and panic disorder in the community. *J Neuropsychiatry Clin Neurosci.* 2007. In press.

12. Salih AM, Gray RE, Mills KR, Webley M. A clinical, serological and neurophysiological study of restless legs syndrome in rheumatoid arthritis. *Br J Rheumatol.* 1994;33:60-63.

13. Gemignani F, Brindani F, Vitetta F, Marbini A, Calzetti S. Restless legs syndrome in diabetic neuropathy: a frequent manifestation of small fiber neuropathy. *J Peripher Nerv Syst.* 2007;12:50-53.

14. Aigner M, Prause W, Freidl M, et al. High prevalence of restless legs syndrome in somatoform pain disorder. *Eur Arch Psychiatry Clin Neurosci.* 2007;257(1):54-57.

15. Lugaresi E, Cirignotta F, Coccagna G, Montagna P. Nocturnal myoclonus and restless legs syndrome. *Adv Neurol.* 1986;43:295-307.

16. Lugaresi E, Coccagna G, Berti-Ceroni G, Ambrosetto C. Restless legs syndrome and nocturnal myoclonus. In: Gastaut H, ed. *The Abnormalities of Sleep in Man.*, Bologna: Aulo Gaggi Editore; 1968:285-294.

17. Zucconi M, Ferri R, Allen R, et al. The official World Association of Sleep Medicine (WASM) standards for recording and scoring periodic leg movements in sleep (PLMS) and wakefulness (PLMW) developed in collaboration with a task force from the International Restless Legs Syndrome Study Group (IRLSSG). *Sleep Med.* 2006;7:175-183.

18. American Academy of Sleep Medicine. *International Classification of Sleep Disorders: Diagnostic and Coding Manual, 2nd Version.* Chicago, IL: American Association of Sleep Medicine; 2005.

19. American Academy of Sleep Medicine. *The AASM Manual for the Scoring of Sleep and Associated Events: Rules, Terminology and Technical Specification.* Westchester, IL: American Association of Sleep Medicine; 2007.

20. Pollmacher T, Schulz H. Periodic leg movements (PLM): their relationship to sleep stages. *Sleep.* 1993;16:572-577.

21. Chabli A, Michaud M, Montplaisir J. Periodic arm movements in patients with the restless legs syndrome. *Eur Neurol.* 2000;44:133-138.

22. Nicolas A, Michaud M, Lavigne G, Montplaisir J. The influence of sex, age and sleep/wake state on characteristics of periodic leg movements in restless legs syndrome patients. *Clin Neurophysiol.* 1999;110:1168-1174.

43

23. Michaud M, Poirier G, Lavigne G, Montplaisir J. Restless Legs Syndrome: scoring criteria for leg movements recorded during the suggested immobilization test. *Sleep Med*. 2001;2:317-321.

24. Ferri R, Zucconi M, Manconi M, et al. Different periodicity and time structure of leg movements during sleep in narcolepsy/cataplexy and restless legs syndrome. *Sleep*. 2006;29:1587-1594.

25. Desautels A, Turecki G, Montplaisir J, Sequeira A, Verner A, Rouleau GA. Identification of a major susceptibility locus for restless legs syndrome on chromosome 12q. *Am J Hum Genet*. 2001;69:1266-1270.

26. Bonati MT, Ferini-Strambi L, Aridon P, Oldani A, Zucconi M, Casari G. Autosomal dominant restless legs syndrome maps on chromosome 14q. *Brain*. 2003;126:1485-1492.

27. Stefansson H, Rye DB, Hicks A, et al. A genetic risk factor for periodic limb movements in sleep. *N Engl J Med*. 2007;357(7):639-647.

28. Birinyi PV, Allen RP, Hening W, Washburn T, Lesage S, Earley CJ. Undiagnosed individuals with first-degree relatives with restless legs syndrome have increased periodic limb movements. *Sleep Med*. 2006;7:480-485.

29. Ancoli-Israel S, Kripke DF, Mason W, Messin S. Sleep apnea and nocturnal myoclonus in a senior population. *Sleep*. 1981;4:349-358.

30. Ancoli-Israel S, Kripke DF, Mason W, Kaplan OJ. Sleep apnea and periodic movements in an aging sample. *J Gerontol*. 1985;40:419-425.

31. Pennestri MH, Whittom S, Adam B, Petit D, Carrier J, Montplaisir J. PLMS and PLMW in healthy subjects as a function of age: prevalence and interval distribution. *Sleep*. 2006;29:1183-1187.

32. Schenck CH, Mahowald MW. Motor dyscontrol in narcolepsy: rapid-eye-movement (REM) sleep without atonia and REM sleep behavior disorder. *Ann Neurol*. 1992;32:3-10.

33. Bahammam A. Periodic leg movements in narcolepsy patients: impact on sleep architecture. *Acta Neurol Scand*. 2007;115:351-355.

34. Schenck CH, Mahowald MW. Polysomnographic, neurologic, psychiatric, and clinical outcome report on 70 consecutive cases with REM sleep behavior disorder (RBD): sustained clonazepam efficacy in 89.5% of 57 cases. *Cleve Clin J Med*. 1990;57(suppl):S9-S23.

35. Fantini ML, Michaud M, Gosselin N, Lavigne G, Montplaisir J. Periodic leg movements in REM sleep behavior disorder and related autonomic and EEG activation. *Neurology*. 2002;59:1889-1894.

36. Montplaisir J, Boucher S, Poirier G, Lavigne G, Lapierre O, Lesperance P. Clinical, polysomnographic, and genetic characteristics of restless legs syndrome: a study of 133 patients diagnosed with new standard criteria. *Mov Disord*. 1997;12:61-65.

37. Michaud M, Paquet J, Lavigne G, Desautels A, Montplaisir J. Sleep laboratory diagnosis of restless legs syndrome. *Eur Neurol*. 2002;48:108-113.

38. Sforza E, Johannes M, Claudio B. The PAM-RL ambulatory device for detection of periodic leg movements: a validation study. *Sleep Med*. 2005;6:407-413.

39. Sforza E, Haba-Rubio J. Night-to-night variability in periodic leg movements in patients with restless legs syndrome. *Sleep Med*. 2005;6:259-267.

40. Mendelson WB. Are periodic leg movements associated with clinical sleep disturbance? *Sleep*. 1996;19:219-223.

41. Carskadon MA, Brown ED, Dement WC. Sleep fragmentation in the elderly: relationship to daytime sleep tendency. *Neurobiol Aging*. 1982;3:321-327.

42. Guilleminault C, Kim YD, Palombini L, Li K, Powell N. Upper airway resistance syndrome and its treatment. *Sleep*. 2000;23(suppl 4):S197-S200.

43. Pennestri MH, Montplaisir J, Colombo R, Lavigne G, Lanfranchi PA. Nocturnal blood pressure changes in patients with restless legs syndrome. *Neurology*. 2007;68:1213-1218.

44. Winkelman JW, Finn L, Young T. Prevalence and correlates of restless legs syndrome symptoms in the Wisconsin Sleep Cohort. *Sleep Med*. 2006;7:545-552.

45. Akpinar S. Treatment of restless legs syndrome with levodopa plus benserazide. *Arch Neurol*. 1982;39:739.

46. Littner MR, Kushida C, Anderson WM, et al. Practice parameters for the dopaminergic treatment of restless legs syndrome and periodic limb movement disorder. *Sleep*. 2004;27:557-559.

47. Vignatelli L, Billiard M, Clarenbach P, et al. EFNS guidelines on management of restless legs syndrome and periodic limb movement disorder in sleep. *Eur J Neurol*. 2006;13:1049-1065.

48. Stiasny-Kolster K, Kohnen R, Moller JC, Trenkwalder C, Oertel WH. Validation of the "L-DOPA test" for diagnosis of restless legs syndrome. *Mov Disord*. 2006;21:1333-1339.

3

Who Gets RLS and How Does It Progress?

Epidemiology of RLS

Restless legs syndrome (RLS) is a common disorder in Western populations. In the last 12 years, there have been several epidemiologic studies that have indicated that RLS symptoms have a prevalence on the order of 5% to 10% in Western countries (European, the United States, some South American countries with strong European roots).[1,2] While these studies have used questionnaires, a recent study using physicians trained in diagnosing RLS found that the prevalence is likely to be at least the low end of this range (5%) (*Richard Allen, personal communication, June 2007*).

Studies of other populations have resulted in highly variable results. Some Asian studies have found a very low prevalence of RLS in the general population (<1%),[3,4] others have found an intermediate level (1% to 4%),[5,6] while still others have found a higher prevalence in the Western population range (5% to 10%).[7,8] One study in South American Indian populations found an intermediate prevalence, higher at altitude.[9] Because of this variability and use of very different protocols to make diagnoses, it is difficult as of yet to make a clear determination of the prevalence in these populations relative to Western ones. This point is underlined by the finding in one population study that prevalence in African Americans was at least as high as that in whites,[10] although clinical practice had suggested a much lower prevalence in African Americans (who rarely were seen for RLS at expert centers).

■ Risk Factors

Table 3.1 summarizes risk factors for RLS identified from different studies. The most important general population risk factors are age and sex.

Age

As illustrated in **Figure 3**.1, the risk of RLS rises with age. Most studies have looked only at adults, but

TABLE 3.1 — Risk Factors for Development of RLS
Demographic Factors • Older age* • Female sex* • Living at higher altitude • Lower socioeconomic status
Lifestyle Factors • Lack of exercise • Smoking
Medical Conditions
General • Pregnancy* • Poor physical health • Poor general health • Obesity
Specific Disorders • Iron deficiency and anemia* • Renal failure* • Polyneuropathy • Diabetes • Parkinson's disease • Multiple sclerosis • Hypothyroidism • Gastric resection • B_{12} deficiency • Spinocerebellar ataxia type 3: Machado-Joseph disease • Lung transplant • Magnesium deficiency
* These are best established risk factors.

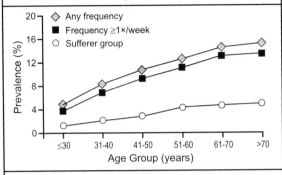

FIGURE 3.1 — RLS Prevalence Figures by Age in the Primary Care REST Study

This figure plots by age in decades the frequency of restless legs syndrome in this population, broken down into groups according to frequency of symptoms. The sufferer group had symptoms at least twice a week and some impact from symptoms when they occurred.

Hening W, et al. *Sleep Med.* 2004;5:237-246.

a recent population study of children indicates that prevalence also rises during the childhood years, with 0.5% of children 8 to 12 and 1.0% of children 13 to 17 having RLS.[11] Some studies have shown that beyond age 65 or 70, there may be a decrease in frequency of RLS. The explanation for this decline is unknown and may relate either to biologic factors or to response factors (the oldest individuals may be less likely to endorse RLS symptoms).

Sex

Women have about twice the risk of developing RLS as men. The figures from some recent studies are given in **Table 3.2**. Two studies have found that RLS is increased in women who have been pregnant; the frequency of RLS in never-pregnant women was not significantly different from that of men.[1,12] In the German

TABLE 3.2 — RLS Symptom Prevalence in Men and Women

Study Author	Location	Overall (%)	Men (%)	Women (%)
Ulfberg 2001 *[1,2]	Sweden	—	5.8	11.4
Sevim 2003[3]	Turkey	3.2	2.5	3.9
Berger 2004[4]	Germany	10.4	7.6	13.4
Allen 2005[5]	Europe-USA	7.2	5.4	9.0
Bjorvatn 2005[6]	Scandinavia	11.5	9.4	13.4
Hogl 2005[7]	Italian Tirol	10.6	6.6	14.2
Kim 2005[8]	Korea	12.1	8.5	15.4
Tison 2005[9]	France	8.5	5.8	10.8

* Ulfberg did separate studies for men and women.

[1]Ulfberg J, et al. *Eur Neurol.* 2001;46:17-19; [2]Ulfberg J, et al. *Mov Disord.* 2001;16:1159-1163; [3]Sevim S, et al. *Neurology.* 2003;61:1562-1569; [4]Berger K, et al. *Arch Intern Med.* 2004;164:196-202; [5]Allen RP, et al. *Arch Intern Med.* 2005;165:1286-1292; [6]Bjorvatn B, et al. *Sleep Med.* 2005;6:307-312; [7]Hogl B, et al. *Neurology.* 2005;64:1920-1924; [8]Kim J, et al. *Psychiatry Clin Neurosci.* 2005;59:350-353; [9]Tison F, et al. *Neurology.* 2005;65:239-246.

study, frequency of RLS also increased with additional pregnancies, so that the risk for women with three or more pregnancies was 3.57 that of men.[1] Pregnancy is also an immediate cause for RLS: between 20% and 25% of pregnant women have RLS, with more than half of them developing the condition for the first time during pregnancy.

Family History

As discussed later, those who are related to RLS patients are more likely to have RLS.

Life Style and Health Issues

Various studies have found that obesity (increased body mass index [BMI]), general poor physical and mental health, and smoking may be related to an increased frequency of RLS symptoms.

Medical Conditions

The most important and well-established conditions are iron deficiency and renal failure.

Medications

Dopamine-receptor–blocking medications and many antidepressants may provoke RLS or aggravate preexisting symptoms.

■ Secondary RLS

The most important conditions that cause RLS are iron deficiency, renal failure, pregnancy, rheumatoid conditions, neuropathy, and diabetes. RLS may also be more common in patients with Parkinson's disease.

Iron Deficiency and Anemia

The finding that iron deficiency can cause RLS goes back to Ekbom; iron therapy was an early treatment studied.[13] In recent years, this association has been confirmed.[14-16] Iron treatment, either oral or intravenous, may benefit RLS. As discussed in Chapter 4, *Pathophysiology*, a deficiency of brain iron is considered a likely cause of at least some RLS. Bleeding conditions, such as caused by nonsteroidal anti-inflammatory medications or cancer, can present with RLS.[17-20]

Renal Failure

Studies have generally found an elevated frequency of RLS in renal patients,[21,22] although this has ranged from a low of 6.6% in India[4] to a high of 70% in Hong Kong, China.[23] There have been no consistent findings of specific factors that predispose to RLS, although this is a population that is, in general, both iron deficient and anemic. More aggressive modern treatment of anemia and iron deficiency with epoetin and intravenous iron may be reducing the frequency, but this has not been well demonstrated.

Pregnancy

Some 20% to 25% of women will have RLS during pregnancy.[24,25] More than half of these women develop RLS for the first time during pregnancy; in most of these with newly developed RLS, symptoms will remit near the time of delivery.

Rheumatoid Conditions

Patients with select rheumatoid conditions, including rheumatoid arthritis,[26] scleroderma,[27] Sjogren's syndrome,[28] and fibromyalgia,[29] may experience increased RLS.

Neuropathy

It has long been suggested that RLS is associated with neuropathy, but one study found only a 5% frequency of RLS in neuropathy patients.[30] Two more recent studies from one group found a clearly increased frequency of RLS in both polyneuropathy[31] and diabetic neuropathy[32] patients.

Diabetes

Most studies have suggested that RLS is more common in diabetes, but only recently has there been a convincing case series indicating that RLS is more frequent in diabetics, perhaps due to the associated neuropathy.[33]

Relationship to Parkinson's Disease

Parkinson's disease (PD) bears an unusual relationship to RLS. On the one hand, the same dopaminergic medications help both conditions. In other ways, they are quite different: Patients with PD have increased iron in the brain; those with RLS, low; PD affects more men; RLS, more women. Some studies have found an increased frequency of RLS,[34] but noted that most RLS began after PD, atypical for familial or idiopathic RLS.

Other Conditions

Other conditions that might cause RLS, some of which are only suggested, are presented in **Table 3.1**.

Genetics of RLS

■ **Familial Aggregation**

Several case series clearly established that more than half of RLS patients are aware of affected relatives.[35-37] This has since been confirmed by formal interview studies that diagnosed relatives directly,[38] clearly showing that patients with idiopathic RLS are more likely to have affected relatives than those with secondary RLS (due to renal failure). A best estimate of the increased risk to first-degree relatives of RLS patients is that they are about five times as likely to have

RLS as are nonrelatives.[39] These studies do indicate that RLS runs in families, but this may be due either to genetics or to a shared common environment.

■ **Segregation Analyses**

One way to sort out genetic and environmental causes is to do a segregation analysis that determines the genetic model that best explains how a disorder runs in a family. Two studies have now shown that the pattern of RLS in a family is that of a dominant inheritance (one abnormal allele determines disease likelihood) in at least some RLS families.[40,41] This supports the likelihood that at least some of the familial aggregation in RLS is genetic. One of the studies also showed that the age at onset is under genetic control.[41]

■ **Linkage and Association Analyses**

Direct genetic studies of RLS identified five suspect locations on five different chromosomes (**Table 3.3**). Near one of these, on 12q, an association has been found to the neuronal nitrogen oxide synthetase gene (NOS1).[42] Recently, two groups have reported associations linked to three specific genes, one confirmed in two studies (2p, 6p, 15q) (**Table 3.3**).[43,44] It is clear that RLS is a complex disorder and that there are a number of genetic and environmental factors that contribute to its causation.

The Clinical Picture of RLS

■ **The Spectrum of Severity**

RLS has a wide variety of severities from rare, nondisturbing episodes that are barely remembered to severe, almost unremitting symptoms that last for most of the day and prevent most of sleep at night. In the community, several studies have suggested that:

- About 15% to 20% have daily or almost daily symptoms
- About 40% have at least weekly, but not daily symptoms
- About 40% have less than weekly symptoms.

The REST studies found that both for patients of a primary physician[45] and for members of the general population,[2] about one third of those identified as having RLS symptoms had symptoms sufficiently severe to merit medical intervention (bothersome symptoms that occur at least twice a week). More recent studies have confirmed using physician diagnosis that this group makes up 1% to 2% of the adult population.

Patients with mild RLS often have symptoms only when they are forced to spend long periods under restrained rest. As RLS worsens, it becomes more frequent and symptoms may be present for longer periods of the day. This is the basis of the Johns Hopkins RLS Severity Scale[46] (**Table 3.4**). In the patients with the most severe RLS, symptoms can be present for most of the day and may only be partially relieved with activity. In some patients, RLS crisis or "status" can occur.[47]

■ **The Course of RLS: RLS Is a Chronic Disorder**
    RLS is almost invariably a chronic condition. In the Hopkins family study, >95% of those diagnosed with idiopathic RLS who had ever had RLS previously continued to have it at the time of interview, for an average duration of almost 20 years. This included many who had quite mild symptoms (less than once a week). Patients with RLS usually describe a progressive course. Those with younger-age onset, most likely to be familial and idiopathic, describe a slowly progressive course; those with later onset, usually secondary, experience a more rapidly progressive course.[48] However, family members, often with milder

TABLE 3.3 — Genetic Linkages and Associations in RLS

Author	Population	Linkage	Model
Linkages			
RLS1—Desautels 2001[1]	French Canadian	12q	Recessive
RLS2—Bonafi 2003[2]	Italian	14q	Dominant
RLS3—Chen 2004[3]	United States	9p	Dominant
RLS4—Levchenko 2006[4]	French Canadian	20p	Dominant
RLS5—Pichler 2006[5]	Italian Tirol	2q	Dominant

Author	Population	Chromosome	Gene
Associations			
Winkelmann et al[6]	French Canadian/European	2p 6p 15q	MEIS1, exon 9 BTBD9, intron 5 MAP2K5, LBXCOR1
Stefannson et al*[7]	Icelandic/United States	6p	BTBD9, intron
Winkelmann et al[8]	European	12q	NOS1

* This association appears to be more related to increased periodic limb movements than to the subjective symptoms of RLS, but the Winkelmann association in the same gene was ascertained in a population defined by subjective symptoms.

[1]Desautels A, et al. *Am J Hum Genet.* 2001;69:1266-1270; [2]Bonati MT, et al. *Brain.* 2003;126:1485-1492; [3]Chen S, et al. *Am J Hum Genet.* 2004;74:876-835; [4]Levchenko A, et al. *Neurology.* 2006;67:900-901; [5]Pichler I, et al. *Am J Hum Genet.* 2006;79:716-723; [6]Winkelmann J, et al. *Nature Genet* 2007;39(8):1000-1006; [7]Stefannson H, et al. *N Engl J Med.* 2007, July 18; Epub ahead of print; [8]Winkelmann J, et al. *Mov Disord.* 2007. Late Breaking Abstracts, page 8.

TABLE 3.4 — The Johns Hopkins RLS Severity Scale	
Occurrence of RLS	**Rating**
No RLS	0
Less than daily RLS	0.5
RLS only beginning at bedtime or in the night	1
RLS beginning after 6 PM but before bedtime	2
RLS beginning before 6 PM	3
RLS beginning before noon	4

symptoms, report that their course is stable or even improving over the years.

This chronicity is important in treating RLS: the doctor has to recognize that this is not a disorder that can be treated acutely and resolved, but like diabetes, hypertension, and cardiovascular disease, is a chronic disorder that will require continued intervention over a span of many years.

RLS in Special Populations

There are additional considerations for diagnosing and managing RLS in special populations. Children can have distinctive features and require more circumspect dosing. Cognitively impaired adults may not be able to provide the key indicia that are necessary to confirm the diagnosis. The character of RLS as manifest in secondary RLS conditions may vary somewhat from the typical picture of idiopathic RLS.

■ RLS in Children
Most adolescents, children ≥12 years of age, are capable of providing a clinical history sufficient to use adult criteria for diagnosing RLS. However, children <12 years of age may not be able to describe their leg

sensations or may give them juvenile terms (such as "owies" or "thingies"); they may be less aware of a circadian factor and most bothered in school, where they may be thought to have attention deficit hyperactivity disorder (ADHD).[49] This led to the 2002 NIH workshop to propose a somewhat more rigorous diagnostic scheme for children,[50] but one which also utilized the supportive criteria of PLMS and family history (**Table 3.5**). In addition, particularly for research purposes, the workshop proposed that diagnosis of probable or possible RLS be considered for children who could not meet full diagnostic criteria (**Table 3.6**). Recent research has made it clear that in the past, children with true RLS may have been mistakenly diagnosed with either ADHD[51,52] or growing pains.[53,54]

■ RLS in the Cognitively Impaired Elderly

This group of patients may be the most difficult to work with since their intellectual, linguistic, and memory functions may not permit an adequate assessment of their RLS features. The 2002 NIH workshop offered some suggestions for how to diagnose these individuals (**Table 3.7**). Ongoing studies are attempting to clarify the diagnostic approach to these patients (*Richard Allen, personal communication, July 12, 2007*). The problem of RLS in this group, especially within closed communities such as nursing homes, is that they may be subject to a variety of factors that can induce or aggravate RLS, including restraint (eg, at night if they are wandering) and the use of provocative medications (eg, dopamine blockers and SSRIs or SNSRIs). It therefore behooves the treating physician to consider the diagnosis when sufficient indicia are present to suggest it; treatment with an RLS-friendly regimen may be better for managing mood and behavior in these patients than major dopamine-blocking tranquilizers or antidepressants. As with all elderly individuals, there must often be caution to avoid pos-

TABLE 3.5 — Diagnosis of RLS in Children (Under Approximately Age 12 Years)

Criteria for the Diagnosis of Definite RLS in Children
Child meets all four of the following adult criteria: 1. An urge to move the legs   2. The urge to move begins or worsens when sitting or lying down   3. The urge to move is partially or totally relieved by movement   4. The urge to move is worse in the evening or night than during the day or only occurs in the evening or night
and
The child uses his or her own words to describe leg discomfort.   Examples of age-appropriate descriptors: owies, tickle, tingle, static, bugs, spiders, ants, boo-boos, want to run, and a lot of energy in my legs.
OR
Child meets all four of the above adult criteria and two or three of the following supportive criteria: 1. Sleep disturbance for age   2. Biological parent or sibling has definite RLS   3. The child has a sleep study documenting a periodic limb movement index of five or more per hour of sleep
Allen RP, et al. *Sleep Med.* 2003;4:101-119.

sible drug interactions in this patient class that is prone to present with polypharmacy.

■ **RLS in Those With Secondary Disorders**

As a general matter, the diagnosis of RLS in secondary disorders usually precedes in the same way as that of idiopathic RLS, but the relationship of the primary condition (cause or mere comorbidity) needs to be defined. The development of one condition before the other or the close temporal relationship between

TABLE 3.6 — Research Diagnosis for Probable or Possible RLS in Children

Criteria for the Diagnosis of Probable RLS in Children

Child meets all four of the following adult criteria except #4:
1. An urge to move the legs
2. The urge to move begins or worsens when sitting or lying down
3. The urge to move is partially or totally relieved by movement
4. The urge to move is worse in the evening or night than during the day or only occurs in the evening or night

and

The child has a biological parent or sibling with definite RLS.

OR

The child is observed to have behavior manifestations of lower-extremity discomfort when sitting or lying, with motor movement of the affected limbs. The discomfort has characteristics of adult criteria 2, 3, and 4 above; worse during rest and inactivity, relieved by movement, and worse during the evening and night.

and

The child has a biological parent or sibling with definite RLS.

Criteria for the Diagnosis of Possible RLS in Children

The child has periodic limb movement disorder.

and

The child has a biologic parent or sibling with definite RLS, but the child does not meet definite or probable childhood RLS definitions.

Allen RP, et al. *Sleep Med.* 2003;4:101-119.

TABLE 3.7 — Diagnosis of RLS in Cognitively Impaired Elderly*

Historical Issues
- History of RLS diagnosed by a medical professional
- Family member's report of typical RLS features
- Affected family members
- Past evidence of a high number of PLMS
- Written evidence in which patient expresses RLS features

Current Observations
- Signs of leg discomfort, such as expressions of pain or attempts to rub, massage, or strike legs
- Excessive motor activity in legs, including fidgeting, shaking, pushing back and forth, twisting, flexing, and extending
- Signs of agitation and inability to stay still, excessive walking
- Inability to get to sleep because of restless activity and exaggerated motor activity during sleep period
- Resistance to restraint or increased signs of discomfort when seated
- Reduced indication of leg discomfort when active, moving, or walking
- Nocturnal accentuation of behavioral signs
- Observed or documents excessive PLM (>25/hour)

Review activity regulations and current medications to determine if RLS-provocative procedures or substances are present

Abbreviations: PLM, periodic limb movements; PLMS, periodic limb movements in sleep

* May be also applied to younger individuals who have cognitive limitations due to developmental issues, disease, or trauma.

Modified from: Allen RP, et al. *Sleep Med.* 2003;4:101-119.

improvement and aggravation of the two conditions are factors that may help determine their relationship. In uremic RLS, it has been shown that PLM are particularly prominent.[55] While the treatment of a causative condition may also benefit RLS, it is often the case that "bridge" or even permanent treatment with RLS-specific medications may be needed to manage the conditions.

REFERENCES

1. Berger K, Luedemann J, Trenkwalder C, John U, Kessler C. Sex and the risk of restless legs syndrome in the general population. *Arch Intern Med*. 2004;164:196-202.

2. Allen RP, Walters AS, Montplaisir J, et al. Restless legs syndrome prevalence and impact: REST general population study. *Arch Intern Med*. 2005;165:1286-1292.

3. Tan EK, Seah A, See SJ, Lim E, Wong MC, Koh KK. Restless legs syndrome in an Asian population: a study in Singapore. *Mov Disord*. 2001;16:577-579.

4. Bhowmik D, Bhatia M, Gupta S, Agarwal SK, Tiwari SC, Dash SC. Restless legs syndrome in hemodialysis patients in India: a case controlled study. *Sleep Med*. 2003;4:143-146.

5. Sevim S, Dogu O, Camdeviren H, et al. Unexpectedly low prevalence and unusual characteristics of RLS in Mersin, Turkey. *Neurology*. 2003;61:1562-1569.

6. Mizuno S, Miyaoka T, Inagaki T, Horiguchi J. Prevalence of restless legs syndrome in non-institutionalized Japanese elderly. *Psychiatry Clin Neurosci*. 2005;59:461-465.

7. Kim J, Choi C, Shin K, et al. Prevalence of restless legs syndrome and associated factors in the Korean adult population: the Korean Health and Genome Study. *Psychiatry Clin Neurosci*. 2005;59:350-353.

8. Rangarajan S, D'Souza GA. Restless legs syndrome in Indian patients having iron deficiency anemia in a tertiary care hospital. *Sleep Med*. 2007;8:247-251.

9. Castillo PR, Kaplan J, Lin SC, Fredrickson PA, Mahowald MW. Prevalence of restless legs syndrome among native South Americans residing in coastal and mountainous areas. *Mayo Clin Proc*. 2006;81:1345-1347.

10. Lee HB, Hening WA, Allen RP, Earley CJ, Eaton WW, Lyketsos CG. Race and restless legs syndrome symptoms in an adult community sample in east Baltimore. *Sleep Med*. 2006;7:642-645.

11. Picchietti D, Allen RP, Walters AS, Davidson JE, Myers A, Ferini Strambi I. Restless legs syndrome: prevalence and impact in children and adolescents, the Peds REST study. *Pediatrics*. 2007;120(2):253-266.

12. Hening WA, Allen RP, Lasage S, Earley CJ. The risk of RLS depends on gender and history of pregnancy in a case-control family study. *Neurology*. 2007;68:A345. Abstract.

13. Nordlander NB. Therapy in restless legs. *Acta Med Scand*. 1953;145:453-457.

14. O'Keeffe ST, Noel J, Lavan JN. Restless legs syndrome in the elderly. *Postgrad Med J*. 1993;69:701-703.

15. O'Keeffe ST, Gavin K, Lavan JN. Iron status and restless legs syndrome in the elderly. *Age Ageing*. 1994;23:200-203.

16. Sun ER, Chen CA, Ho G, Earley CJ, Allen RP. Iron and the restless legs syndrome. *Sleep*. 1998;21:371-377.

17. Leutgeb U, Martus P. Regular intake of non-opioid analgesics is associated with an increased risk of restless legs syndrome in patients maintained on antidepressants. *Eur J Med Res*. 2002;7:368-378.

18. Ekbom KA. Restless legs as an early symptom of cancer. *Sven Lakartidn*. 1955;52:1875-1883.

19. Brocklehurst J. Restless legs syndrome as a presenting symptom in malignant disease. *Age Ageing*. 2003;32:234.

20. Morcos Z. Restless legs syndrome, iron deficiency and colon cancer. *J Clin Sleep Med*. 2005;1:433.

21. Winkelman JW, Chertow GM, Lazarus JM. Restless legs syndrome in end-stage renal disease. *Am J Kidney Dis*. 1996;28:372-378.

22. Kavanagh D, Siddiqui S, Geddes CC. Restless legs syndrome in patients on dialysis. *Am J Kidney Dis*. 2004;43:763-771.

23. Hui DS, Wong TY, Li TS, et al. Prevalence of sleep disturbances in Chinese patients with end stage renal failure on maintenance hemodialysis. *Med Sci Monit*. 2002;8:CR331-CR336.

24. Manconi M, Govoni V, De Vito A, et al. Restless legs syndrome and pregnancy. *Neurology*. 2004;63:1065-1069.

25. Tunc T, Karadag YS, Dogulu F, Inan LE. Predisposing factors of restless legs syndrome in pregnancy. *Mov Disord*. 2007;22:627-631.

26. Salih AM, Gray RE, Mills KR, Webley M. A clinical, serological and neurophysiological study of restless legs syndrome in rheumatoid arthritis. *Br J Rheumatol*. 1994;33:60-63.

27. Prado GF, Allen RP, Trevisani VM, Toscano VG, Earley CJ. Sleep disruption in systemic sclerosis (scleroderma) patients: clinical and polysomnographic findings. *Sleep Med*. 2002;3:341-345.

28. Gudbjornsson B, Broman JE, Hetta J, Hallgren R. Sleep disturbances in patients with primary Sjogren's syndrome. *Br J Rheumatol*. 1993;32:1072-1076.

29. Yunus MB, Aldag JC. Restless legs syndrome and leg cramps in fibromyalgia syndrome: a controlled study. *BMJ*. 1996;312:1339.

30. Rutkove SB, Matheson JK, Logigian EL. Restless legs syndrome in patients with polyneuropathy. *Muscle Nerve*. 1996;19:670-672.

31. Gemignani F, Brindani F, Negrotti A, Vitetta F, Alfieri S, Marbini A. Restless legs syndrome and polyneuropathy. *Mov Disord*. 2006;21:1254-1257.

32. Gemignani F, Brindani F, Vitetta F, Marbini A, Calzetti S. Restless legs syndrome in diabetic neuropathy: a frequent manifestation of small fiber neuropathy. *J Peripher Nerv Syst*. 2007;12:50-53.

33. Lopes LA, Lins Cde M, Adeodato VG, et al. Restless legs syndrome and quality of sleep in type 2 diabetes. *Diabetes Care*. 2005;28:2633-2636.

34. Ondo WG, Vuong KD, Jankovic J. Exploring the relationship between Parkinson disease and restless legs syndrome. *Arch Neurol*. 2002;59:421-424.

35. Walters AS, Hickey K, Maltzman J, et al. A questionnaire study of 138 patients with restless legs syndrome: the 'Night-Walkers' survey. *Neurology*. 1996;46:92-95.

36. Ondo W, Jankovic J. Restless legs syndrome: clinicoetiologic correlates. *Neurology*. 1996;47:1435-1441.

37. Montplaisir J, Boucher S, Poirier G, Lavigne G, Lapierre O, Lesperance P. Clinical, polysomnographic, and genetic characteristics of restless legs syndrome: a study of 133 patients diagnosed with new standard criteria. *Mov Disord*. 1997;12:61-65.

38. Winkelmann J, Wetter TC, Collado-Seidel V, et al. Clinical characteristics and frequency of the hereditary restless legs syndrome in a population of 300 patients. *Sleep*. 2000;23:597-602.

39. Allen RP, La Buda MC, Becker P, Earley CJ. Family history study of the restless legs syndrome. *Sleep Med*. 2002;3(suppl):S3-S7.

40. Winkelmann J, Muller-Myhsok B, Wittchen HU, et al. Complex segregation analysis of restless legs syndrome provides evidence for an autosomal dominant mode of inheritance in early age at onset families. *Ann Neurol*. 2002;52:297-302.

41. Mathias RA, Hening W, Washburn M, et al. Segregation analysis of restless legs syndrome: possible evidence for a major gene in a family study using blinded diagnoses. *Hum Hered*. 2006;62:157-164.

42. Winkelmann J, Lichtner P, Schormair B, et al. Variants in the neuronal nitric oxide synthase (nNOS, NOS1) gene are associated with restless legs syndrome (abstr). *Mov Disord*. 2007. Late Breaking Abstracts: p. 8.

3

43. Winkelmann J, Schormair B, Lichtner P, et al. Genome-wide association study in restless legs syndrome identifies common variants in three genomic regions. *Nature Genet.* 2007;39(8):1000-1006.

44. Stefansson H, Rye DB, Hicks A, et al. A genetic risk factor for periodic limb movements in sleep. *N Engl J Med.* 2007, July 18. Epub ahead of print.

45. Hening W, Walters AS, Allen RP, Montplaisir J, Myers A, Ferini-Strambi L. Impact, diagnosis and treatment of restless legs syndrome (RLS) in a primary care population: the REST (RLS epidemiology, symptoms, and treatment) primary care study. *Sleep Med.* 2004;5:237-246.

46. Allen RP, Earley CJ. Validation of the Johns Hopkins restless legs severity scale. *Sleep Med.* 2001;2:239-242.

47. Vahedi H, Kuchle M, Trenkwalder C, Krenz CJ. Peridural morphine administration in restless legs status. *Anasthesiol Intensivmed Notfallmed Schmerzther.* 1994;29:368-370.

48. Allen RP, Earley CJ. Defining the phenotype of the restless legs syndrome (RLS) using age-of-symptom-onset. *Sleep Med.* 2000;1:11-19.

49. Picchietti DL, England SJ, Walters AS, Willis K, Verrico T. Periodic limb movement disorder and restless legs syndrome in children with attention-deficit hyperactivity disorder. *J Child Neurol.* 1998;13(12):588-594.

50. Allen RP, Picchietti D, Hening WA, Trenkwalder C, Walters AS, Montplaisi J; Restless Legs Syndrome Diagnosis and Epidemiology workshop at the National Institutes of Health; International Restless Legs Syndrome Study Group. Restless legs syndrome: diagnostic criteria, special considerations, and epidemiology. A report from the restless legs syndrome diagnosis and epidemiology workshop at the National Institutes of Health. *Sleep Med.* 2003;4(2):101-119.

51. Walters AS, Picchietti DL, Ehrenberg BL, Wagner ML. Restless legs syndrome in childhood and adolescence. *Pediatr Neurol.* 1994;11(3):241-245.

52. Cortese S, Konofal E, Lecendreux M, et al. Restless legs syndrome and attention-deficit/hyperactivity disorder: a review of the literature. *Sleep.* 2005;28(8):1007-1013.

53. Walters AS. Is there a subpopulation of children with growing pains who really have Restless Legs Syndrome? A review of the literature. *Sleep Med.* 2002;3(2):93-98.

54. Rajaram SS, Walters AS, England SJ, Mehta D, Nizam F. Some children with growing pains may actually have restless legs syndrome. *Sleep.* 2004;27(4):767-773.

55. Wetter TC, Stiasny K, Kohnen R, Oertel WH, Trenkwalder C. Polysomnographic sleep measures in patients with uremic and idiopathic restless legs syndrome. *Mov Disord.* 1998;13(5):820-924.

4

Pathophysiology

Nervous System Dysfunction

Restless legs syndrome (RLS) is generally considered to be a disorder arising from the central nervous system (CNS), even though no specific lesion has been found. Due to the absence of any evident neurodegeneration or cell loss and the preservation of most other CNS capabilities, it is likely that RLS represents a functional, rather than a structural, abnormality. There is some evidence for RLS-related alterations at all levels of the neuraxis, from spinal cord to cortex, and even a suggestion that, at least in some patients, abnormalities of peripheral nerves may contribute to development of RLS (**Table 4.1**).

■ **Electrophysiologic Studies**

While not all studies are positive, several studies have suggested that there might be enhanced reflex activity in RLS, especially increases in late components of reflexes. This has been found for spinal flexion reflexes in both primary[1] and secondary RLS[2] and for startle reflexes (mediated by the reticulospinal tract).[3] Transcranial magnetic stimulation studies have found intact motor pathways, but evidence for decreased intracortical and subcortical inhibition, suggesting hyperexcitation due to diminished inhibition.[4-7] These alterations can be reversed by dopaminergic therapy.[8]

■ **Imaging Studies**

General studies of brain structure[9] and resting metabolism[10] have found no abnormalities in RLS. One functional magnetic resonance imaging (fMRI) study

TABLE 4.1 — Evidence for Involvement of Different Regions of the Nervous System in RLS

Peripheral Nerves
- Increased evidence of neuropathy in RLS patients[1,2]

Spinal Cord
- Presence of PLM in cord transected patients[3]
- Abnormal spinal reflexes in RLS[4]

Brainstem
- Abnormal reticular formation and red nucleus activation during symptoms[5,6]

Cerebellum
- Abnormal cerebellar activation during symptoms[5]

Thalamus
- Increased pulvinar gray matter density[7]

Basal Ganglia
- Autopsy studies show iron deficiency and protein abnormalities in substantia nigra[8,9]
- MRI and echo show reduced brainstem iron in RLS[10-13]

Cortex
- Imaging evidence of abnormal status of cortical pain areas[6,14]
- Magnetic stimulation demonstrates decreased intracortical inhibition[15,16]

Abbreviations: MRI, magnetic resonance imaging; PLM, periodic limb movement.

[1]Iannaccone S, et al. *Mov Disord.* 1995;10:2-9; [2]Polydefkis M, et al. *Neurology.* 2000;55:1115-1121; [3]de Mello MT, et al. *Spinal Cord.* 1996;34:294-296; [4]Bara-Jimenez W, et al. *Mov Disord.* 1998;13(suppl 2):294; [5]Bucher SF, et al. *Ann Neurol.* 1997;41:639-645; [6]von Spiczak S, et al. *Brain.* 2005;128:906-917; [7]Etgen T, et al. *Neuroimage.* 2005;24:1242-1247; [8]Wang X, et al. *J Neurol Sci.* 2004;220:59-66; [9]Connor JR, et al. *Neurology.* 2003;61:304-309; [10]Allen RP, et al. *Neurology.* 2001;56:263-265; [11]Earley CJ, et al. *Sleep Med.* 2006;7:458-461; [12]Schmidauer C, et al. *Ann Neurol.* 2005;58:630-634; [13]Godau J, et al. *Mov Disord.* 2007;22:187-192; [14]San Pedro EC, et al. *J Rheumatol.* 1998;25:2270-2275; [15]Tergau FS, et al. *Neurology.* 1999;53:861-864; [16]Scalise A, et al. *Sleep.* 2006;29:770-775.

found abnormal bilateral cerebellar and thalamic activation during sensory symptoms, with additional red nucleus and reticular formation activity during periodic limb movements in wake (PLMW).[9] A single-photon emission computed tomography (SPECT) study of an affected parent/child pair showed changes consistent with pain (decreased caudate and increase anterior cingulate blood flow).[11] A positron emission tomography (PET) study using an opioid ligand found that there was altered activity in brain regions associated with the medial pain system (especially orbitofrontal cortex and anterior cingulate).[12] One MRI study found bilateral increases in gray matter in the pulvinar nucleus of the thalamus,[13] but this was not confirmed in drug-naïve subjects.[14] Dopamine-related imaging studies are discussed later.

■ Circadian Rhythms

The overall circadian rhythm is regulated by the suprachiasmatic nucleus of the hypothalamus, keeping many body functions cycling within a period of around 24 hours.[15,16] It has been established that all RLS symptoms also have a circadian rhythm with peak activity between the late evening and early morning (approximately 21:00 to 4:00 hours).[17-19] This period largely coincides with the daily rise in melatonin secretion, a key biologic marker of the intrinsic circadian clock.[20] The link between melatonin and RLS is not clear, but may represent merely multiple effects of a general circadian process or might indicate some specific influence of melatonin on RLS.

In summary, a variety of studies have suggested that while no discrete CNS lesion has been found in RLS, there may be altered function at various levels of the CNS. The peripheral nervous system may also influence the development or expression of symptoms. However, these studies have not yet revealed what is the key locus or loci in causing RLS. There may, however, be more clues from examining altered neurotransmitter and metabolic systems in RLS.

Neurotransmitter Systems

■ **Dopamine and CNS Iron**

The connection of RLS to the dopamine system has been established by the response of RLS to dopaminergic treatments in almost all studies performed to date. After the initial studies reported the response of RLS to levodopa and a dopamine agonist,[21-23] the idea developed that RLS, like Parkinson's disease, might be a disorder with decreased brain dopamine stores and possible neurodegeneration. Some imaging studies supported a decrease in dopamine markers,[24] but others found only normal values.[25] The most recent imaging study reported that D_2 dopamine receptors were increased both within and without the striatum.[26] The authors of those study results argued that this provided evidence for a decreased function of dopamine presynaptically. Another possible abnormality concerning dopamine could be an altered amplitude of its circadian rhythm.[27-29] Cerebrospinal fluid (CSF) studies have found that dopamine metabolites show greater circadian variation in RLS patients than in controls.[30] RLS patients may have as much dopamine as others—perhaps even more at certain phases of the daily cycle—but the variation may induce symptoms selectively at certain times of day. This effect may explain one endocrine study that found that administered levodopa selectively produced enhanced endocrine responses when administered to patients in the evening.[31]

One hypothesis that may provide a mechanism for such dopamine abnormalities is the idea that in many cases, RLS is induced by inadequate levels of CNS iron.[32-34] Several lines of evidence for this concept are listed in **Table 4.2**. The basic hypothesis (**Figure 4.1**)

TABLE 4.2 — Evidence for the Iron-Dopamine Hypothesis for Causation of RLS

Iron Deficiency Is Associated With RLS

Prominent Secondary RLS Conditions Are Associated With Iron Deficiency
- Pregnancy
- Anemia
- Uremia
- Rheumatoid arthritis

CSF Findings
- RLS patients show decreased CSF levels of iron storage marker (ferritin) and increased transferrin
- RLS patients show strong circadian rhythm of dopamine metabolites and related compounds[1]

Brain Iron Levels
- *In vivo* studies show low brainstem iron
- Autopsy studies show low levels of iron in substantia nigra neurons with decreased ferritin and increased transferrin[2]
- Autopsy studies show abnormalities of iron regulating proteins consistent with decreased transferrin receptor in the face of low iron[3]

Altered Dopamine-System Autopsy Findings in Iron Deficient RLS Patients
- Decreased thy-1 synaptic adhesion protein
- Increased tyrosine hydroxylase, dopamine, and dopamine metabolites

Animal Models
- A11 spinal dopamine tract lesion creates rodents with behavioral similarities to RLS[4]
- Feeding iron-deficient diet enhances RLS-like behaviors[5]

Abbreviation: CSF, cerebrospinal fluid.

[1]Earley CJ, et al. *Sleep Med.* 2006;7:263-268; [2]Connor JR, et al. *Neurology.* 2003;61:304-309; [3]Connor JR, et al. *Neurology.* 2004;62:1563-1567; [4]Clemens S, et al. *Neurology.* 2006;67:125-130; [5]Ondo WG, et al. *Sleep Med.* 2007;8:344-348.

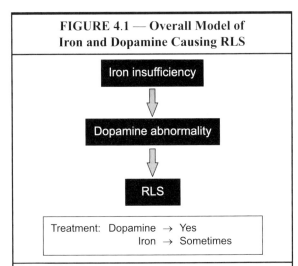

FIGURE 4.1 — Overall Model of Iron and Dopamine Causing RLS

Iron insufficiency

Dopamine abnormality

RLS

Treatment: Dopamine → Yes
Iron → Sometimes

The model stresses that the primary deficit is in reduced iron levels that then cause abnormalities in dopamine-system functioning. A major support for the hypothesis is the therapeutic benefit obtained regularly with dopamine and sometimes with iron supplementation.

is that either through altered cellular mechanisms or depressed body stores, the iron levels in dopaminergic neurons drop (**Figure 4.2**). As a consequence, neuronal function changes and the result may be disruption of synaptic function[35] or accentuation of the circadian rhythm of dopamine.[36] Under this concept, those with familial, genetically based RLS may have a tendency toward depressed uptake and retention of brain iron, while those with secondary RLS may often have conditions in which body iron stores are depleted, thereby drawing out iron from the brain. While this model is highly promising, key details remain to be elucidated and the role of this mechanism for inducing RLS needs to be established. Studies of brain iron deficiencies in humans with RLS have focused on the substantia nigra, the key nucleus for parkinsonian pathology.

FIGURE 4.2 — Midbrain Stained for Iron in RLS Patient and Control

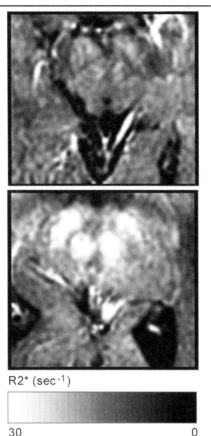

R2* (sec⁻¹)

30   0

R2* magnetic resonance images in a 70-year-old, RLS patient *(top)* and a 71-year-old, control subject *(bottom)*. Much lower R2* relaxation rates are apparent in the RLS case in both red nucleus and substantia nigra, indicating lower iron content.

Allen RP, et al. *Neurology*. 2001;56:263-265.

However, voluntary motor function is normal in most RLS patients.[37] Animal-model studies have generally concentrated on the A11 dopamine system, a diffuse and hard-to-study cell grouping that sends dopaminergic axons down to the spinal cord.[38] To date, it has not been conclusively shown that disrupting the A11 system produces a suitable model for RLS, and studies on the human A11 system have not been done. We are therefore still unsure which dopaminergic system is most responsible for RLS.

Other Systems

The endogenous opiate system has been implicated in RLS by the favorable response of patients to a wide variety of opioid medications.[39-42] Imaging studies have also suggested that RLS symptoms are correlated with activity or binding changes in pain-relevant CNS structures.[11,12] One early case study provided some evidence that RLS might act through the dopamine system,[43] but strong opioids have been found to be effective even when dopamine agents have failed or have caused iatrogenic exacerbation of RLS (augmentation).[42] Reversal of therapeutic effect by opioid blockers (naloxone) does indicate that the effect is specific to the endogenous opiate system.[44] The exact role of opioids and the relation between the opiate and dopamine systems remain areas for further exploration.

Other neuronal systems—the adrenergic, serotoninergic, glutaminergic, gabaergic, orexinergic, histaminergic, and adenosinergic—have been implicated by some therapeutic or other studies in RLS, but evidence for and understanding of their potential roles is only at an early stage. Given the complex interrelationships of neural systems in the brain, it is likely that many systems may play some role in modulating the development, expression, and perception of RLS symptoms.

REFERENCES

1. Bara-Jimenez W, Hallett M. Increased spinal cord excitability in patients with restless legs syndrome. *Mov Disord.* 1998;13(suppl 2):294.

2. Aksu M, Bara-Jimenez W. State dependent excitability changes of spinal flexor reflex in patients with restless legs syndrome secondary to chronic renal failure. *Sleep Med.* 2002;3:427-430.

3. Frauscher B, Loscher WN, Hogl B, Poewe W, Kofler M. Auditory startle reaction is disinhibited in idiopathic restless legs syndrome. *Sleep.* 2007;30:489-493.

4. Tergau F, Wischer S, Paulus W. Motor system excitability in patients with restless legs syndrome. *Neurology.* 1999;52:1060-1063.

5. Stiasny-Kolster K, Haeske H, Tergau F, Muller HH, Braune HJ, Oertel WH. Cortical silent period is shortened in restless legs syndrome independently from circadian rhythm. *Suppl Clin Neurophysiol.* 2003;56:381-389.

6. Scalise A, Cadore IP, Gigli GL. Motor cortex excitability in restless legs syndrome. *Sleep Med.* 2004;5:393-396.

7. Scalise A, Pittaro-Cadore I, Golob EJ, Gigli GL. Absence of postexercise and delayed facilitation of motor cortex excitability in restless legs syndrome: evidence of altered cortical plasticity? *Sleep.* 2006;29:770-775.

8. Nardone R, Ausserer H, Bratti A, et al. Cabergoline reverses cortical hyperexcitability in patients with restless legs syndrome. *Acta Neurol Scand.* 2006;114:244-249.

9. Bucher SF, Seelos KC, Oertel WH, Reiser M, Trenkwalder C. Cerebral generators involved in the pathogenesis of the restless legs syndrome. *Ann Neurol.* 1997;41:639-645.

10. Trenkwalder C, Walters AS, Hening WA, et al. Positron emission tomographic studies in restless legs syndrome. *Mov Disord.* 1999;14:141-145.

11. San Pedro EC, Mountz JM, Mountz JD, Liu HG, Katholi CR, Deutsch G. Familial painful restless legs syndrome correlates with pain dependent variation of blood flow to the caudate, thalamus, and anterior cingulate gyrus. *J Rheumatol.* 1998,25.2270-2275.

12. von Spiczak S, Whone AL, Hammers A, et al. The role of opioids in restless legs syndrome: an [11C]diprenorphine PET study. *Brain.* 2005;128:906-917.

13. Etgen T, Draganski B, Ilg C, et al. Bilateral thalamic gray matter changes in patients with restless legs syndrome. *Neuroimage.* 2005;24:1242-1247.

14. Hornyak M, Ahrendts JC, Spiegelhalder K, et al. Voxel-based morphometry in unmedicated patients with restless legs syndrome. *Sleep Med.* 2007 May 17. Epub ahead of print.

15. Saper CB, Lu J, Chou TC, Gooley J. The hypothalamic integrator for circadian rhythms. *Trends Neurosci.* 2005;28:152-157.

16. Schibler U. Circadian time keeping: the daily ups and downs of genes, cells, and organisms. *Prog Brain Res.* 2006;153:271-282.

17. Hening WA, Walters AS, Wagner M, et al. Circadian rhythm of motor restlessness and sensory symptoms in the idiopathic restless legs syndrome. *Sleep.* 1999;22:901-912.

18. Trenkwalder C, Hening WA, Walters AS, Campbell SS, Rahman K, Chokroverty S. Circadian rhythm of periodic limb movements and sensory symptoms of restless legs syndrome. *Mov Disord.* 1999;14:102-110.

19. Michaud M, Dumont M, Paquet J, Desautels A, Fantini ML, Montplaisir J. Circadian variation of the effects of immobility on symptoms of restless legs syndrome. *Sleep.* 2005;28:843-846.

20. Michaud M, Dumont M, Selmaoui B, Paquet J, Fantini ML, Montplaisir J. Circadian rhythm of restless legs syndrome: relationship with biological markers. *Ann Neurol.* 2004;55:372-380.

21. Akpinar S. Treatment of restless legs syndrome with levodopa plus benserazide. *Arch Neurol.* 1982;39:739.

22. Montplaisir J, Godbout R, Poirier G, Bedard MA. Restless legs syndrome and periodic movements in sleep: physiopathology and treatment with L-dopa. *Clin Neuropharmacol.* 1986;9:456-463.

23. Walters AS, Hening WA, Kavey N, Chokroverty S, Gidro-Frank S. A double-blind randomized crossover trial of bromocriptine and placebo in restless legs syndrome. *Ann Neurol.* 1988;24:455-458.

24. Turjanski N, Lees AJ, Brooks DJ. Striatal dopaminergic function in restless legs syndrome: 18F-dopa and 11C-raclopride PET studies. *Neurology.* 1999;52:932-937.

25. Eisensehr I, Wetter TC, Linke R, et al. Normal IPT and IBZM SPECT in drug-naive and levodopa-treated idiopathic restless legs syndrome. *Neurology.* 2001;57:1307-1309.

26. Cervenka S, Palhagen SE, Comley RA, et al. Support for dopaminergic hypoactivity in restless legs syndrome: a PET study on D2-receptor binding. *Brain.* 2006;129:2017-2028.

27. Davila R, Zumarraga M, Andia I, Friedhoff AJ. Persistence of cyclicity of the plasma dopamine metabolite, homovanillic acid, in neuroleptic treated schizophrenic patients. *Life Sci.* 1989;44:1117-1121.

28. Doran AR, Pickar D, Labarca R, et al. Evidence for a daily rhythm of plasma HVA in normal controls but not in schizophrenic patients. *Psychopharmacol Bull*. 1985;21:694-697.

29. Kawano Y, Kawasaki T, Kawazoe N, et al. Circadian variations of urinary dopamine, norepinephrine, epinephrine and sodium in normotensive and hypertensive subjects. *Nephron*. 1990;55:277-282.

30. Earley CJ, Hyland K, Allen RP. Circadian changes in CSF dopaminergic measures in restless legs syndrome. *Sleep Med*. 2006;7:263-268.

31. Garcia-Borreguero D, Larrosa O, Granizo JJ, de la Llave Y, Hening WA. Circadian variation in neuroendocrine response to L-dopa in patients with restless legs syndrome. *Sleep*. 2004;27:669-673.

32. Earley CJ, Allen RP, Beard JL, Connor JR. Insight into the pathophysiology of restless legs syndrome. *J Neurosci Res*. 2000;62:623-628.

33. Allen RP, Earley CJ. The role of iron in restless legs syndrome. *Mov Disord*. 2007 June 12. Epub ahead of print.

34. Allen R. Dopamine and iron in the pathophysiology of restless legs syndrome (RLS). *Sleep Med*. 2004;5:385-391.

35. Wang X, Wiesinger J, Beard J, et al. Thy1 expression in the brain is affected by iron and is decreased in Restless Legs Syndrome. *J Neurol Sci*. 2004;220:59-66.

36. Dean T Jr, Allen RP, O'Donnell CP, Earley CJ. The effects of dietary iron deprivation on murine circadian sleep architecture. *Sleep Med*. 2006;7:634-640.

37. Alberts JL, Adler CH, Saling M, Stelmach GE. Prehension patterns in restless legs syndrome patients. *Parkinsonism Relat Disord*. 2001;7:143-148.

38. Clemens S, Rye D, Hochman S. Restless legs syndrome: revisiting the dopamine hypothesis from the spinal cord perspective. *Neurology*. 2006;67:125-130.

39. Walters AS, Wagner ML, Hening WA, et al. Successful treatment of the idiopathic restless legs syndrome in a randomized double-blind trial of oxycodone versus placebo. *Sleep*. 1993;16:327-332.

40. Walters AS, Winkelmann J, Trenkwalder C, et al. Long-term follow-up on restless legs syndrome patients treated with opioids, *Mov Disord*. 2001;16:1105-1109.

41. Vignatelli L, Billiard M, Clarenbach P, et al. EFNS guidelines on management of restless legs syndrome and periodic limb movement disorder in sleep. *Eur J Neurol*. 2006;13:1049-1065.

42. Ondo WG. Methadone for refractory restless legs syndrome. *Mov Disord*. 2005;20:345-348.

43. Montplaisir J, Lorrain D, Godbout R. Restless legs syndrome and periodic leg movements in sleep: the primary role of dopaminergic mechanism. *Eur Neurol*. 1991;31:41-43.

44. Walters A, Hening W, Cote L, Fahn S. Dominantly inherited restless legs with myoclonus and periodic movements of sleep: a syndrome related to the endogenous opiates? *Adv Neurol*. 1986;43:309-319.

5

Consequences

Restless legs syndrome (RLS) has a myriad of consequences, especially for patients with moderate to severe symptoms. The most significant consequence tends to be its impact on sleep. The sleep disruption caused by RLS creates many other problems. In addition, several other unique aspects of this disease create havoc in the life of RLS sufferers.

Impact on Sleep

■ Difficulty Getting to Sleep

Bedtime tends to be a difficult time for patients with moderate to severe RLS. The bothersome symptoms are typically peaking at this time and can easily prevent people from falling asleep. Upon going to bed, symptoms tend to dramatically increase, forcing sufferers to move their affected limbs or get out of bed and walk. Patients with RLS often refer to themselves as "night walkers," which is also the name given to the quarterly newsletter published by the RLS Foundation.

The REST General Population Study[1] (which interviewed >16,000 adults in the United States, France, Germany, Italy, Spain, and the UK) found that 75.5% of the RLS sufferers (people reporting moderately to severely distressing RLS symptoms at least twice weekly) reported at least one sleep-related symptom. About 48% of these RLS sufferers reported an inability to fall asleep.

The REST Primary Care Study[2] (which investigated >23,000 patients from the practices of 182 primary care physicians in the United States, France,

Germany, Spain, and the UK) found that 68.6% of RLS sufferers (people with RLS symptoms at least twice weekly with an appreciable negative impact on their quality of life) took 30 minutes or longer to fall asleep (**Figure 5.1**).

Unlike people with other medical problems who cannot fall asleep, those not sleeping due to RLS cannot simply go to another bed or a comfortable place to try to fall asleep or even rest. People with milder and intermittent forms of RLS may not have significant problems falling asleep. They may report occasional difficulty falling asleep but, in general, sleep is not a major issue with this group. However, for severe cases, their RLS symptoms force them to move their legs (and other affected body parts) turning them into the earlier-mentioned night walkers. This has been described as torture, especially when it recurs night after night and may last for hours.

Many of those who have their RLS symptoms relieved by treatment find that they continue to have problems falling asleep. After years of disrupted sleeping patterns due to RLS symptoms, sufferers may develop abnormal sleeping patterns, such as being conditioned not to fall asleep at bedtime. Therefore, it is not unusual to have to treat them for persistent insomnia even after the RLS symptoms have been completely resolved.

■ Difficulty in Maintaining Sleep

The REST primary care study[2] also showed that RLS sufferers have difficulty maintaining sleep. They found that 60.1% of this group woke up three or more times per night (**Figure 5.2**). Upon awakening, it may be very difficult for such RLS sufferers to fall back asleep due to their bothersome RLS symptoms. Sleep deprivation from the inability to fall asleep and maintain sleep can be considerable and often results in further daytime consequences as discussed below.

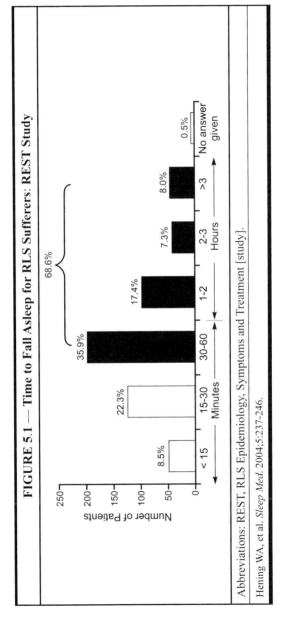

FIGURE 5.1 — Time to Fall Asleep for RLS Sufferers: REST Study

Abbreviations: REST, RLS Epidemiology, Symptoms and Treatment [study].

Hening WA, et al. *Sleep Med.* 2004;5:237-246.

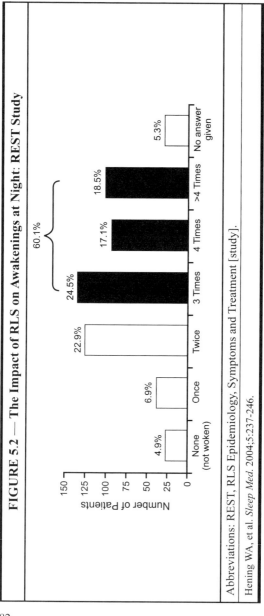

FIGURE 5.2 — The Impact of RLS on Awakenings at Night: REST Study

Abbreviations: REST, RLS Epidemiology, Symptoms and Treatment [study].

Hening WA, et al. *Sleep Med.* 2004;5:237-246.

Impact on Daytime Function

The effect of sleep deprivation from both sleep-onset and sleep-maintenance insomnia described above can be substantial. When combined with the inability to rest during the daytime (for those with more severe RLS) due to RLS symptoms, these people can have significant disruptions in their lifestyle and daily activities.

■ Fatigue and Daytime Sleepiness

The REST primary care study[2] found that 60.1% of RLS sufferers reported that they lacked energy when experiencing RLS symptoms and 57.2% of this group stated that their daily activities were disturbed. Another study[3] found that 61% of RLS patients studied had increased sleepiness assessed by the Epworth Sleepiness Scale and increased fatigue assessed by Fatigue Severity Scale. Furthermore, the above studies and an additional one in 2004[4] found RLS sufferers to have a decrease in their energy/vitality scores on the Short Form 36 Health Survey (SF-36). One recent study even demonstrated that increased daytime sleepiness was dose related to more frequent RLS symptoms.[5] On occasion, the inability to sleep at nighttime may be so severe that the patient may walk most of the night or fall asleep only while standing. This somnambulant behavior presents health and safety risks exemplified by one case report about a patient whose RLS resulted in repeated falls causing multiple skeletal fractures.[6]

Complaints of daytime fatigue are very common in RLS sufferers. Despite battling these symptoms, many do try to lead full, normal lives. The problem of sleepiness would be expected to result in an increase in motor vehicle accidents, which does not yet appear to be the case. It may be that bothersome RLS symptoms, which tend to increase while driving may prevent the onset of sleep. For the same reason, it is often difficult for people with RLS to nap during the daytime despite their sleep deprivation.

- ■ **Concentration and Cognition**
    The sleep deprivation described can account for significant problems with concentration and cognition. The resulting fatigue, coupled with the intrusion of bothersome RLS symptoms, provides understanding of the impairment experienced by RLS patients. Not many studies have yet examined this issue, but the REST general population study found that 19.2% of RLS sufferers reported difficulty concentrating in the afternoon, and 17.5%, the next evening after not sleeping well.

    A recent study[7] that specifically examined cognitive deficits associated with moderate to severe RLS found similar sizeable deficits, especially with verbal fluency, to those reported losing a full night of sleep. The cognitive tests were done in the morning (when RLS symptoms are usually absent) to assess the affects of sleep disruption in RLS subjects. The ability to concentrate and think would most likely have been markedly worse if these tests had been done in the late afternoon or evening when RLS symptoms are more prevalent. The influence of these significant decreases in cognitive function and concentration on daily life is discussed below.

Impact on Mood

Many studies have found high prevalence of depression and anxiety symptoms in RLS patients.[1-5,8-9] It is not yet completely clear whether this association is due to a symptomatic epiphenomenon or shared pathophysiological mechanism between RLS and mood disorder. However, most RLS experts believe that depression and anxiety are strongly associated and frequently co-occur among RLS patients. Complicating this issue is that many of the drugs used to treat depression and anxiety tend to worsen RLS. The relationship between RLS and both depression and anxiety is explored in greater detail in Chapter 12, *RLS and Psychiatric Disorders*.

It is thought that the chronic discomfort of RLS symptoms (similar to that of any other chronic pain disorder) and chronic insomnia lead to depression.[10] As noted, the association of depression and RLS has been made repeatedly in the medical literature. One recent study demonstrated a dose relationship between RLS symptoms frequency and self-reported depression and anxiety outcomes.[5]

As noted, it is not yet clearly determined if RLS symptoms cause depression. One recent study[9] found that most patients developed their anxiety or depression after the onset of RLS symptoms, suggesting that depression may occur because of the RLS symptoms.

Impact on General Health

Several recent studies have demonstrated a marked decrease in general health in people with RLS.[1-4,8] The SF-36 scores in these studies reveal significantly decreased quality of life very similar to that of other chronic disorders (such as depression, chronic obstructive pulmonary disease, osteoarthritis, diabetes, congestive heart failure, etc). In addition, the general health, bodily pain, and physical functioning role parameters are universally decreased. This disease has a marked impact on the life of RLS patients.

One recent study[5] found a cross-sectional association of RLS symptoms with cardiovascular disease similar to that in a previous study in Sweden.[11] The cause of this association may be similar to that of other sleep disorders such as sleep apnea that involve an increase in cardiovascular disease. One study found an increase in hypertension in RLS patients,[12] but this was not confirmed in another population-based study.[13]

Thus far, it does not seem that RLS has an effect on longevity. Despite the many years of suffering, people with the disorder have been known to live to >100 years of age.

Avocational Impairment

RLS can easily prevent people from enjoying many of the social pleasures in life. All sedentary situations are troublesome, and those that also prevent movement are often completely avoided.

■ Social Events

Religious services, social meetings (eg, book clubs, lectures), and evenings with friends or family are often on the list of things to be avoided. The more formal situations such church services are especially difficult as movement or walking are clearly not appropriate. However, even in the less-formal setting of a family get-together, it may be difficult to repeatedly justify the seemingly strange movements or walking (while others are sitting) behavior.

In addition, the fatigue, sleepiness, and inability to concentrate that are so common with this disorder may interfere with the ability to attend and enjoy these events. Therefore, many RLS sufferers simply shun them and keep making up excuses (usually not related to their strange RLS problems that most do not understand) in order not go at all.

In one respect, theater and movies pose less of a threat in that the anonymity associated with them is somewhat protective. Excuses and explanations may have to be given briefly to strangers rather than to close friends or relatives. However, the long sedentary duration involved make them extremely difficult for people with RLS. Many who merely experience rare bedtime symptoms will find RLS symptoms preventing them from enjoying and seeing the end of these shows.

Some coping mechanisms may enable those with RLS to go to the movies or theater. Sitting in an aisle seat or on the back row may facilitate movement or going for a quick walk to relieve symptoms. It may be possible to walk and view the performance from behind a glass at the back of the auditorium. However, many RLS patients feel that the effort and stigma of relieving their symptoms in public are just not worth it and tend to avoid these venues.

5

Relationships With Friends and Family

Relationships tend to be a problem for those with significant RLS problems. The restrictions placed upon those with the disorder often prevent them from forming and maintaining close relationships.

■ Family and Friends

The relationships that are made with family and friends are often sustained by sharing common activities, such as watching TV, going to movies or church, sitting and talking while at meals, travel, etc. Of course, these sedentary activities limit the ability of an RLS patient to participate. To add to the problem, those with RLS may be quite fatigued and lack the energy to even join active events that would not bother their RLS.

Even though it may be apparent that the person really wants to participate in such events, their family and friends tend to get tired of hearing the repeated excuses and may assume that the person does not want to socialize with them. Many RLS patients feel isolated and will avoid their friends and family. The anxiety and depression that are more common with this disorder tend to further restrict their ability to bond with others.

People with RLS become frustrated with their friends and family as they hear over and over again,

"But you don't look like you have a medical condition; you look well enough to go out with us tonight!" As the RLS symptoms do not have any serious-appearing external manifestations (except for the person walking, rubbing the affected area of leg, kicking), this disorder is usually not taken very seriously by friends and family. The excuse of RLS is often interpreted as just not wanting to be with or do things with the friends and family members.

■ **Intimacy (Spousal/Bed Partner Issues)**

Dating can be a problem as described above with forming relationships with friends. However, becoming intimate and sharing a bed presents even more difficulties. Bedtime is when RLS symptoms tend to peak, thereby making it very difficult to rest in bed. The spouse or bed partner can easily get annoyed at the continued movements necessary to relieve RLS symptoms. Once asleep, the periodic limb movements (PLM) may disturb the bed partner or even cause them injury.

Not being able to sleep with the bed partner is often misconstrued as not wanting to sleep with them and easily results in hurt feeling. There are many anecdotal reports of this leading to the breakup of couples or marriages. The loss of the ability to share a bed with your partner is one of the major complaints of those afflicted with RLS. It is bad enough that they must endure the isolation due to difficulties of maintaining relationships with family and friends, but in addition, they may lose the intimacy and support of their spouse or partner.

Occupational Consequences

Just as RLS impacts other facets of daily life, work is similarly affected. Any occupation that requires sedentary activities is prone to be problematic. Often, these impediments to performing a job can be worked around. However, many types of employment are not as flexible and may thus not be suitable for those with RLS.

■ Impact on Job Performance and Selection

Any occupation that includes desk work, long meetings, driving long distances, or other sedentary tasks is stressful for most RLS patients. This clearly encompasses the vast majority of workplaces, which narrows down the scope of work that is suitable for people with RLS.

That does not mean that anyone developing RLS must quit their job once they develop symptoms while working. There are often ways to work around the problem (discussed later) that may help the person sustain good job performance. Cooperation of fellow employees and management is usually helpful and necessary. It is easy to imagine how a patient with moderate to severe RLS may not be able to sit long hours at a desk or sit with peers or clients during long meetings.

The choice of career may be important to people with RLS. If daytime RLS symptoms keep interfering with performance despite treatment, a different type of job may be preferred. For example, a nurse or schoolteacher may do well despite RLS as their work is conducive to walking whenever necessary and has only a small sedentary component. However, being promoted to administration with the associated desk work and meetings may be a career-ending change.

Shift work may also be problematic for some and may work for others. If the work is not sedentary, it may be appropriate even for the peak RLS hours as long as it allows for adequate sleep time. RLS patients who do not get enough sleep (which is common among shift workers) will develop more problems with their RLS. Shift work should be avoided unless it meets the requirements noted above.

Some people with RLS prefer to be self-employed as they can then choose their hours, the amount of sedentary work, and even change their work environment to adjust to their unique requirements.

Even with an RLS-friendly job, the performance of those with RLS may be have poor. As noted, fatigue, daytime sleepiness, and problems with concentration and thinking may easily impair job performance. Problems with anxiety and depression may further impair the individual from functioning at work and interacting effectively with their coworkers. Inadequate treatment of RLS may easily result in poor job ratings, decreased income, and even loss of employment. Furthermore, some of the drugs used for RLS may cause daytime sleepiness and despite helping RLS may result in impairing work performance.

■ Disability

Those suffering from severe RLS may not be able to adjust adequately to maintain their employment. It is easy to understand that someone who wakes up and cannot even sit down to eat breakfast due to RLS symptoms may not be able to function at any job that requires them to be sedentary. In addition, even for those who have occupations that do not require them to be sedentary, the problems discussed related due to fatigue, daytime sleepiness, decreased concentration and mentation, anxiety, and depression might prevent them from working.

Thus it may be very appropriate for some people with severe RLS to go on disability. Obtaining disability, even for those with more accepted and traditional illnesses, is often difficult. RLS presents additional hurdles as there is no listing for this disorder (by the Social Security Administration or other organizations) and the medical personnel who assess the level of disability generally are not familiar with it. Therefore, the disability must be filed under the resultant consequence of RLS rather than the disorder itself.

If the RLS and PLM are causing excessive daytime sleepiness, objective measures, such as an overnight sleep study, multiple sleep latency test, or maintenance of wakefulness test, may be helpful objective tests to document the degree of disability. Physicians can be instrumental in helping the RLS patient obtain approval for their disability. Proper documentation of the nature and extent of the disability can be critical in such cases. Although many people with disability eventually obtain approval, the process can take a long time. People with RLS have received disability benefits after careful documentation by their health care providers.

Impact on Travel

In our modern fast-paced world, we all take travel for granted. Even people with more typical disabilities (eg, those who are wheelchair bound) have few, if any, problems traveling, as special accommodations for them are now required. The most difficult situation for people with RLS is long airplane trips. Once the seatbelt sign illuminates (for take-off, turbulent weather, etc), there is simply no way to walk off the symptoms, which usually rapidly increase due to the compelled sitting and the resultant increased anxiety. There are some methods of treating this problem that will be discussed in the chapters on treating RLS.

When possible, other modes of transportation are preferable. Trains are better tolerated as one can get up and walk whenever necessary. Buses are somewhat more problematic as there is only a little aisle space in which to walk. Travel by boat should be fine, but that presents only limited opportunities.

Automobile trips are often feasible as long as frequent stops are made for walks. Longer trips can be harder or even impossible for those with more severe RLS.

REFERENCES

1. Allen RP, Walters AS, Montplaisir J, et al. Restless legs syndrome prevalence and impact: REST general population study. *Arch Intern Med.* 2005;165:1286-1292.

2. Hening W, Walters AS, Allen RP, Montplaisir J, Myers A, Ferini-Strambi L. Impact, diagnosis and treatment of restless legs syndrome (RLS) in a primary care population: the REST (RLS epidemiology, symptoms, and treatment) primary care study. *Sleep Med.* 2004;5:237-246.

3. Gerhard R, Bosse A, Uzun D, Orth M, Kotterba S. Quality of life in restless legs syndrome. Influence of daytime sleepiness and fatigue. *Med Klin* (Munich). 2005;100:704-709. German.

4. Abetz L, Allen R, Follet A, et al. Evaluating the quality of life of patients with restless legs syndrome. *Clin Ther.* 2004;26:925-935.

5. Winkelman JW, Finn L, Young T. Prevalence and correlates of restless legs syndrome symptoms in the Wisconsin Sleep Cohort. *Sleep Med.* 2006;7:545-552.

6. Kuzniar TJ, Silber MH. Multiple skeletal injuries resulting from uncontrolled restless legs syndrome. *J Clin Sleep Med.* 2007;3:60-61.

7. Pearson VE, Allen RP, Dean T, Gamaldo CE, Lesage SR, Earley CJ. Cognitive deficits associated with restless legs syndrome (RLS). *Sleep Med.* 2006;7:25-30.

8. Picchietti D, Winkelman JW. Restless legs syndrome, periodic limb movements in sleep, and depression. *Sleep.* 2005;28:891-898.

9. Winkelmann J, Prager M, Lieb R, et al. "Anxietas tibiarum". Depression and anxiety disorders in patients with restless legs syndrome. *J Neurol.* 2005;252:67-71.

10. Breslau N, Roth T, Rosenthal L, Andreski P. Sleep disturbance and psychiatric disorders: a longitudinal epidemiological study of young adults. *Biol Psychiatry.* 1996;39:411-418.

11. Ulfberg J, Nystrom B, Carter N, Edling C. Prevalence of restless legs syndrome among men aged 18 to 64 years: an association with somatic disease and neuropsychiatric symptoms. *Mov Disord.* 2001;16:1159-1163.

12. Rothdach AJ, Trenkwalder C, Haberstock J, Keil U, Berger K. Prevalence and risk factors of RLS in an elderly population: the MEMO study. Memory and Morbidity in Augsburg Elderly. *Neurology.* 2000;54:1064-1068.

13. Sevim S, Dogu O, Camdeviren H, et al. Unexpectedly low prevalence and unusual characteristics of RLS in Mersin, Turkey. *Neurology.* 2003;61:1562-1569.

6

Diagnosis and Evaluation

Diagnosis of restless legs syndrome (RLS) proceeds along the lines suggested in Chapter 2, *Diagnosis and Differential Diagnosis*: taking the history from the patient to determine if the four diagnostic features of RLS are present and probing to be sure that the patient is not describing a mimic. **Table 6.1** outlines the steps to complete the initial evaluation. A recent review covers many of the diagnostic and assessment instruments.[1]

Diagnostic Instruments

A number of diagnostic instruments have been developed for RLS. For screening purposes, a single question has proved useful; it identifies almost all individuals with RLS of any degree and is not answered positively by the majority of individuals.[2,3] The question is: When you try to relax in the evening or sleep at night, do you ever have unpleasant, restless feelings in your legs that can be relieved by walking or movement?

This question cannot accurately diagnose RLS: Depending on the setting, only 25% to 66% of those who answer "yes" will be found to have RLS. A positive response to this screener must be followed by a series of diagnostic questions. Two sets of questions have been validated and are more specific (**Table 6.2** and **Table 6.3**). These questions have generally been used for epidemiologic studies and can be answered by the patient without assistance.

For a more definitive diagnosis, the Hopkins Telephone Diagnostic Interview (HTDI) is a structured set of questions to both diagnose RLS and determine

TABLE 6.1 — Initial Work-Up of RLS

History
- To elucidate symptoms and exclude mimics
- Information on sleep and nighttime motor activity from patient and bed partner or observer
- Review of systems to determine possible causes of

Physical
- Primarily to find possible mimic disorders, causes of RLS, or comorbid conditions that might shape therapy
- Close examination of legs and associated neurologic exam most important

Laboratory
- Blood tests for iron status should be done (ferritin, TIBC, % saturation)
- Screen for anemia, diabetes, and renal failure
- Other blood tests only on clinical suspicion
- Electrodiagnostic tests only if there is suspicion of nerve damage
- Polysomnography (sleep study) not routinely indicated, but may be needed if diagnosis is difficult or an additional sleep disorder suspected
- Suggested immobilization tests or actigraphic monitoring of leg activity may be useful adjuncts

Abbreviation: TIBC, total iron binding capacity.

certain elements of its course. It has been validated and found to be quite accurate but requires specific training for optimal use.[4]

Sleep Diaries

Sleep diaries can be used to chart the occurrence of RLS symptoms and the time of sleep (**Figure 6.1**). They can cover different time periods, but plotting hourly for 5 days to 2 weeks can reveal the frequency and time of day of symptoms as well as their impact on sleep. This can be helpful in determining the timing of medication doses as well as ascertaining how well a treatment is

TABLE 6.2 — Epidemiologic Questionnaire for RLS

Answers to the first three questions should be either YES or NO:

1. Do you have unpleasant sensations (culturally specific descriptor examples) in your legs combined with an urge or need to move your legs?
2. Do these feelings/symptoms occur mainly or only at rest and do they improve with movement?
3. Are these feelings/symptoms worse in the evening or night than in the morning?
4. How often do these feelings/symptoms occur?
   A. <Once/year
   B. At least once a year but <once/month
   C. Once a month
   D. 2 to 4 times/month
   E. 2 to 3 times/week
   F. 4 to 5 times/week
   G. 6 to 7 times/week

Diagnosis of RLS requires a YES answer to the first three questions.

Berger K, et al. *J Neurol.* 2002;249:1195-1199; Allen RP, et al. *Sleep Med.* 2003;4:101-119.

working. Electronic diaries are available that can be combined with actigraphy, although these are usually reserved for basic research or therapeutic studies.

The Medical Outcome Scales for Sleep (MOS) can also provide a subjective assessment for the period of sleep and sleep satisfaction.[5,6] A similar instrument, the Pittsburgh Sleep Quality Index, can also be used to examine aspects of sleep quality.[7,8]

Rating Scales for RLS

The Johns Hopkins Rating Scale (**Table 6.4**)[9] judges severity by the time of symptom onset. Because it is designed to differentiate those with daily or near-

TABLE 6.3 — Validated Patient-Completed Questionnaire

1. Do you have, or have you had, recurrent uncomfortable feelings or sensations in your legs while you are sitting or lying down?	☐ Yes ☐ No
2. Do you have, or have you had, a feeling of a recurrent need or urge to move your leg while you were sitting or lying down?	☐ Yes ☐ No
If you answered YES to either question, continue with Question 3; otherwise STOP.	
3. Are these feelings *always* due to muscle cramps?	☐ Yes ☐ No, they are *not always* due to cramps ☐ Don't know
NOTE: If you answered NO or DON'T KNOW to Question 3, then answer the rest of the questions ONLY for those feelings that are NOT muscle cramps.	
4. Are you more likely to have these feelings when you are resting (either sitting or lying down) or when you are physically active?	☐ Resting ☐ Active
5. If you get up and move around when you have these feelings, do these feelings get any better while you actually keep moving?	☐ Yes ☐ No ☐ Don't know

6. Which times of day are these feelings in your legs most likely to occur? (*Please mark all that apply, ie, one or more than one*)	☐ Morning ☐ Evening ☐ Mid-day ☐ Night ☐ Afternoon ☐ About equal at all times
7. When you actually experience the feelings in your legs, how *distressing* are they?	☐ Not at all distressing ☐ A little bit distressing ☐ Moderately distressing ☐ Extremely distressing
8. In the past 12 months, how often did you experience these feelings in your legs? (*Please mark only one answer*)	☐ Every day ☐ 2 days/month ☐ 4-6 days/week ☐ 1 day/month ☐ 2-3 days/week ☐ <1 day/month ☐ 1 day/week ☐ Never
9. Approximately how old were you when you first noticed these feelings in your legs? (*Please write age*)	_____ Years of age

Diagnosis depends on questions 1 through 6. Questions 7 through 9 provide a basic characterization of the disorder. To have definite RLS, you must answer YES to Questions 1 and 2, YES or Don't Know to 3, Resting to 4, YES to 5, and 6 should include evening and night, although in very severe cases other times may be mentioned. Persons who answer NO to Question 1, but answer the remainder of the questions consistent with RLS may be diagnosed as probable RLS.

Nichols DA, et al. *Sleep.* 2003;36(suppl):A346.

6

FIGURE 6.1 — Example of a Sleep Diary in a Patient With Severe RLS

		Mid-day/Noon			Afternoon				Evening				Midnight						Morning					
DATE	DAY	12-1	1-2	2-3	3-4	4-5	5-6	6-7	7	8	9	10	11	12-1	1-2	2-3	3-4	4-5	5-6	6-7	7	8	9	10	11
	Monday	r	r	R	R	R	R	R	R	R	R	R	V	R	R	R	R	↘	↗	↘	r	r	r	r	r
	Tuesday	•	•	•	r	r	r	R	R	r	R	R	V½	R	R	R	R	R	↘	↘	↗	•	•	•	•
1/26/00	Wednesday	•	•	•	•	r	•	r	•	•	r	R	V½	R	R	R	R	↗	↘ R	↗	r	•	•	•	•
1/27/00	Thursday	•	•	↘	r	•	r	r	•	r	R	•	r	R	R	R	R	↘ R	•	•	•	•	•	•	•
1/28/00	Friday	•	•	•	•	•	r	•	•	•	R	r	r	R	R	r	↘	↗	•	•	•	•	•	•	•
1/29/00	Saturday	•	•	•	r	•	r	•	•	•	•	r	r	r	R	↗	↘	↗	r	•	•	•	•	•	•
1/30/00	Sunday	•	•	•	•	r	•	•	•	•	•	•	•	R	R			↗	•	r	•	•			
1/31/00	Monday	•	Dosing with iron																						
	Tuesday																								

Symptoms are marked for each hour of the day; R = restless legs during the hour; small r for mild or little amount of RLS; capital R for disturbing amount). The patient also marks when going to bed (↓) and when rising (↑). Time spent actually asleep is filled in; part way into a block indicates part way into the hour. A letter code indicates any sleep-related medication taken and in what hour.

Sample courtesy of the RLS Center, Johns Hopkins Bayview Medical Center, Baltimore, MD.

TABLE 6.4 — Johns Hopkins Restless Legs Syndrome Rating Scale (JHRLSS)	
No restless legs syndrome (RLS)	0
Less than almost daily	0.5
Symptoms at bedtime or during sleep	1
Symptoms begin after 18:00 but before bedtime	2
Symptoms begin before 18:00	3
Symptoms begin before noon	4
Before applying, a diagnosis of RLS must be made and the rating applied strictly to RLS symptoms.	
Allen RP, et al. *Sleep Med.* 2001;2:239-242.	

6

daily symptoms, it is less useful for evaluating the severity of milder cases of RLS.

The International RLS Study group rating scale (Appendix A) has been one of the most used primary outcome measures in RLS therapeutic trials. It has been validated and has been found to have excellent psychometric properties.[10-13] The scale measures both the symptoms of RLS and also the impact on sleep, daytime function, mood, and daily activities. It can be seen as having two main factors: symptoms and impact,[14] with sleep bridging the two.[13,15]

The Clinical Global Impression[16] is a summary measure that is used by the treating clinician to assess the condition of the patient (**Table 6.5**). It can be used as a quick way of measuring RLS, although it is a flexible tool that can be applied to many disorders. It has also been used as an important outcome measure in many therapeutic trials. There is also a patient variant of the measure, which is then called a Patient Global Impression, and follows the same form but has the rating assigned by the patient, rather than the clinician.

The RLS-6 Scales (**Table 6.6**) have been used primarily in Europe. These scales ask about the sever-

TABLE 6.5 — Clinical Global Impression (CGI)
CGI—Severity of Illness (CGI-S) • 7-point scale from 1 = not at all ill through 7 = severely ill
CGI—Improvement or Change (CGI-I) • 7-point scale ranging from –3 = very much improved through 0 = unchanged to 3 = very much worse
CGI—Therapeutic Improvement • 4-point scale from 1 = very good (much or very much improved) to 4 = unchanged or worse
CGI—Tolerability (adverse events) • 4-point scale from 1 = no adverse events to 4 = adverse events outweigh benefits
The first two scales, CGI-S and CGI-I, are the ones most used in clinical trials. The Patient Global Impression follows the same format and scoring, but the judgment is made by the patient rather than the clinician or investigator.

ity of RLS symptoms in different situations and times of day, as well as a global sleep assessment. These are visual analogue scales in which the individual assigns a point along a continuum to the degree of current symptoms in each setting. As to be expected, the scales asking about nighttime and sleep are the most heavily endorsed by patients as more bothersome.

Quality of Life

An important concomitant of RLS is an impaired quality of life (QOL). Some studies of RLS have used the SF-36, a standard, general measure of QOL in eight physical and psychological domains,[17] to assess RLS QOL. It has been shown that quality of life is impaired in RLS and that quality decreases with greater severity of RLS (**Figure 6.2**).[18-20] This decrease in those with significant RLS (twice or greater per week and bothersome symptoms) is comparable to chronic

TABLE 6.6 — RLS-6 Scales

Each scale is a visual analogue scale in which the patient or subject places a mark at the point on a (usually) 10-cm line that is marked into 10 segments. The score is determined by measurement of the mark with distance converted into an 11-point 0-to-10 score, where 0 indicates no relevant symptoms/complaints and 10 is the most severe.

1. RLS symptoms at bedtime
2. RLS symptoms during the night
3. RLS symptoms at rest during the daytime
4. RLS symptoms when active during the daytime
5. Satisfaction with sleep
6. Daytime fatigue and tiredness

The first two items tend to show the greatest symptoms, while the fourth item is usually rated very low.

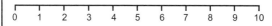

medical conditions such as type 2 diabetes. There are now also two RLS-specific QOL scales targeted at the consequences of RLS symptoms and sleep loss. The RLS quality of life instrument (RLS-QOL) is factored into four domains (daily function, social function, sleep quality, and emotional well-being) and has been validated and found to have good psychometric qualities.[21] The RLS QOL Questionnaire provides a single measure of disorder impact and has also been validated.[22]

Physical Examination

As indicated in **Table 6.1**, the major purpose of the physical examination in RLS is to search for causative or comorbid conditions or to make findings to help with the differential diagnosis. Particular attention should be paid to the legs, with evaluation of any lesions, joint abnor-

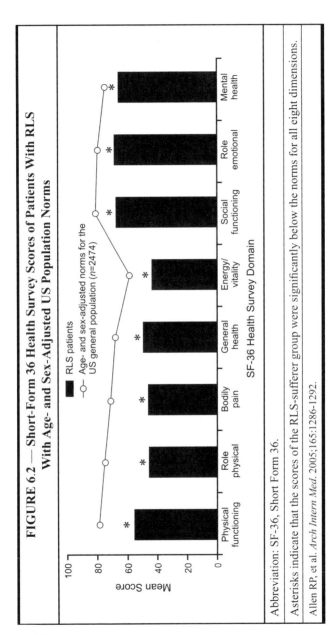

FIGURE 6.2 — Short-Form 36 Health Survey Scores of Patients With RLS With Age- and Sex-Adjusted US Population Norms

Abbreviation: SF-36, Short Form 36.

Asterisks indicate that the scores of the RLS-sufferer group were significantly below the norms for all eight dimensions.

Allen RP, et al. *Arch Intern Med.* 2005;165:1286-1292.

malities, venous engorgement, or decreased pulse. The neurologic exam should determine if there is any loss of sensation in the various modalities and check reflexes and muscle strength, primarily to look for polyneuropathy, radiculopathy, or mononeuropathy. Other aspects of the physical exam may also suggest a systemic process that may be important for assessment.

Laboratory Evaluation

The one obligatory laboratory assessment is to check for iron status, using ferritin (a measure of body iron stores), total binding capacity, and percent saturation. The measurement of iron itself is generally not useful. The presence of ferritin <50 mcg/L should raise considerations of therapeutic iron repletion and levels <30 mcg/L should be followed by a work-up for iron deficiency. Percent saturation <20% has a similar implication. In patients who develop significant treatment resistance or have a sudden deterioration, a follow-up test may reveal newly developed iron deficiency. It must be remembered, however, that ferritin is also an acute-phase reactant, so it should not be measured during any acute illness.

A complete blood count can help find anemia, which may be associated with iron deficiency. Screening for diabetes (blood glucose or glycosylated hemoglobin) or uremia (BUN, creatinine) may be helpful. Other screening for possible causes, such as B_{12} deficiency or autoimmune factors (eg, suggesting rheumatoid arthritis) has not proved useful[23] and should only be pursued when there is some additional reason to suspect such disorders (ie, history or findings on physical exam).

Electrodiagnostic studies to assess nerve function should also be restricted to those who show clear signs of nerve dysfunction (sensory loss, atrophy, weakness) or have a history of progressive numbness or weakness, either generalized or in a restricted distribution. The relationship of RLS to nerve dysfunction is unclear. Much of the nerve dysfunction in RLS involves small fibers whose integrity is not evaluated by standard nerve conduction tests or electromyography.[24-26] In any case, RLS treatment is not much altered by these findings, although there may be some greater preference for using an anticonvulsant such as gabapentin.[26,27]

The polysomnogram (PSG) or sleep study is a standard means of assessing sleep (**Table 6**.7). It measures the length and depth of sleep, the time it takes to get to sleep, and the number of arousals and awakenings. Respiration is measured to determine if there are any sleep-related respiratory disorders. In most studies, leg muscle activity is measured with an EMG to record motor activity, including periodic limb movements (PLMs). Typical abnormal findings from RLS are indicated in **Table 6**.8. These, however, are not considered diagnostic; the American Academy of Sleep Medicine standards indicate that a PSG is not necessary for the routine diagnosis of RLS.[28] Those situations in which a PSG might be useful in RLS include cases of uncertain diagnosis, cases where another sleep disorder is suspected, and cases where treatment with the usual RLS medications has not been helpful.

The suggested immobilization test (SIT) (**Table 2**.3) can be combined with the PSG to gain a clearer picture of RLS. The SIT is performed immediately before the PSG begins, later in the evening (eg, 22:00), since sensory discomfort increases as the time advances towards midnight (**Figure 6**.3). As time goes on, this test may prove to be more important in assessing therapies, especially those aimed at intermittent symptoms.

Actigraphy, as discussed in *Chapter 2*, can be used to gain a more extended picture of sleep continuity and PLM than the PSG. Actigraphic measurement of activity, either over 24 hours or at night, can provide

TABLE 6.7 — The Polysomnogram (Sleep Study)

State Measurement—
These can provide measures of latency to sleep onset and quantity of sleep, different sleep stages (REM and NREM), stage shifts, wakenings, arousals:
- EEG recording: usually at least two leads, one central (C3-A2) and one occipital (O2-A1)
- Eye movement recording: electro-oculogram to measure movement in eyes
- Chin EMG to measure brachial muscle tone

Respiratory Measurement—
This can detect breathing effort and any cessations of breathing (apnea) or diminution (hypopnea). Nasal cannula can determine excess breathing effort (upper airway resistance syndrome):
- Belts to record thoracic and abdominal breathing effort
- Thermistor to record nasal and buccal airflow or nasal cannula to measure pressure
- Oximeter to measure oxygen saturation

Movement Activity—
These can record PLM; in conjunction with mentalis EMG and artifacts on EEG traces, these can indicate generalized movement:
- Bilateral anterior tibialis EMG

Cardiac Measurement
- EKG

Abbreviations: EEG, electroencephalogram; EKG, electrocardiogram; EMG, electromyelogram; NREM, non–rapid eye movement; PLM, periodic limb movements; REM, rapid-eye movement.

Special studies looking for movement disorders or epilepsy may require additional EEG and/or EMG channels.

useful information for shaping treatment. Actigraphy can also be combined with sleep diaries, either paper or electronic, to associate symptom level with motor activity and sleep.

TABLE 6.8 — Typical RLS Findings on a Sleep Study

Sleep States
- Prolonged sleep latency (wake before sleep onset)
- Increased arousals and awakenings
- Increased wake during the night (wake after sleep onset)
- Increased light sleep (non–rapid eye movement stage 1)

Respiratory
- Nothing typical, but RLS can be associated with sleep related breathing disorders[1]

Movement Activity
- Increased periodic limb movements in sleep (usually >5/hour, typically >15/hour)
- Increased periodic limb movements in wake
- Restlessness recorded as generalized movements (epochs scored as movement time)

Cardiac
- Nothing typical, but RLS can be associated with cardiac disorders that may be reflected in abnormal rhythms

[1]Lakshminarayanan S, et al. *Mov Disord.* 2005;20:502-503.

REFERENCES

1. Kohnen R, Allen RP, Benes H, et al. Assessment of restless legs syndrome. Methodological approaches for use in practice and clinical trials. *Mov Disord.* 2007 May 29; Epub ahead of print.
2. Ferri R, Lanuzza B, Cosentino FH, et al. A single question for the rapid screening of restless legs syndrome in the neurological clinical practice. *Eur J Neurol.* 2007;14(9):1016-1021.
3. Hening WA, Sharon D, Abraham M, et al. Validation of a single question screener question for the Restless Legs Syndrome. *Mov Disord.* 2006;21(suppl):S443. Abstract.
4. Hening W, Washburn M, Allen R, Lesage S, Earley C. Validation of the Hopkins telephone diagnostic interview for the restless legs syndrome. *Sleep Med.* 2007 July 16; Epub ahead of print.
5. Stewart AL, Hays RD, Ware JE Jr. The MOS short-form general health survey. Reliability and validity in a patient population. *Med Care.* 1988;26:724-735.

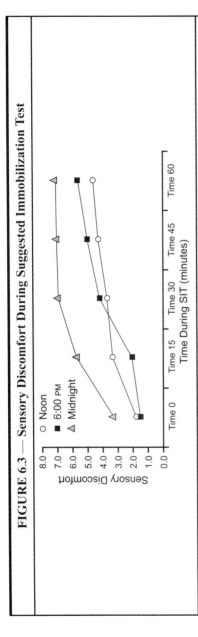

FIGURE 6.3 — Sensory Discomfort During Suggested Immobilization Test

Legend:
○ Noon
■ 6:00 PM
△ Midnight

Y-axis: Sensory Discomfort (8.0, 7.0, 6.0, 5.0, 4.0, 3.0, 2.0, 1.0, 0.0)

X-axis: Time During SIT (minutes) — Time 0, Time 15, Time 30, Time 45, Time 60

Abbreviation: SIT, suggested immobilization test.

This presents data from 11 subjects who had SITs performed at 3-hour intervals with intervening activity. The SITs lasted 60 minutes and sensory discomfort from RLS was rated at the beginning of the SIT and every 15 minutes thereafter. Discomfort was rated on a visual analogue scale of 10 cm running from 0 (no symptoms) to 10 (most severe symptoms possible).

Data reported is based on: Hening WA, et al. *Sleep.* 1999;22:901-912.

107

6. Cunningham WE, Hays RD, Burton TM, Kington RS. Health status measurement performance and health status differences by age, ethnicity, and gender: assessment in the medical outcomes study. *J Health Care Poor Underserved.* 2000;11:58-76.

7. Cole JC, Motivala SJ, Buysse DJ, Oxman MN, Levin MJ, Irwin MR. Validation of a 3-factor scoring model for the Pittsburgh sleep quality index in older adults. *Sleep.* 2006;29:112-116.

8. Backhaus J, Junghanns K, Broocks A, Riemann D, Hohagen F. Test-retest reliability and validity of the Pittsburgh Sleep Quality Index in primary insomnia. *J Psychosom Res.* 2002;53:737-740.

9. Allen RP, Earley CJ. Validation of the Johns Hopkins restless legs severity scale. *Sleep Med.* 2001;2:239-242.

10. Walters AS, LeBrocq C, Dhar A, et al; International Restless Legs Syndrome Study Group. Validation of the International Restless Legs Syndrome Study Group rating scale for restless legs syndrome. *Sleep Med.* 2003;4:121-132.

11. Garcia-Borreguero D, Larrosa O, de la Llave Y, Granizo JJ, Allen R. Correlation between rating scales and sleep laboratory measurements in restless legs syndrome. *Sleep Med.* 2004;5:561-565.

12. Wunderlich GR, Evans KR, Sills T, et al. An item response analysis of the international restless legs syndrome study group rating scale for restless legs syndrome. *Sleep Med.* 2005;6:131-139.

13. Abetz L, Arbuckle R, Allen RP, et al. The reliability, validity and responsiveness of the International Restless Legs Syndrome Study Group rating scale and subscales in a clinical-trial setting. *Sleep Med.* 2006;7:340-349.

14. Allen RP, Kushida CA, Atkinson MJ; RLS QoL Consortium. Factor analysis of the International Restless Legs Syndrome Study Group's scale for restless legs severity. *Sleep Med.* 2003;4:133-135.

15. Kushida CA, Allen RP, Atkinson MJ. Modeling the causal relationships between symptoms associated with restless legs syndrome and the patient-reported impact of RLS. *Sleep Med.* 2004;5:485-488.

16. National Institute of Mental Health, CGI. Clinical global impressions. In: Guy W, ed. *ECDEU Assessment Manual for Psychopharmacology.* Rockville, MD: National Institute of Mental Health; 1976:218-222.

17. Ware JE. SF-36 *Health Survey—Manual and Interpretation Guide.* Boston, MA: Massachusetts Health Institute, New England Medical Center; 1993.

18. Allen RP, Walters AS, Montplaisir J, et al. Restless legs syndrome prevalence and impact: REST general population study. *Arch Intern Med.* 2005;165:1286-1292.

19. Kushida C, Martin M, Nikam P, et al. Burden of restless legs syndrome on health-related quality of life. *Qual Life Res*. 2007;16:617-624.

20. Abetz L, Allen R, Follet A, et al. Evaluating the quality of life of patients with restless legs syndrome. *Clin Ther*. 2004;26:925-935.

21. Atkinson MJ, Allen RP, DuChane J, Murray C, Kushida C, Roth T; RLS Quality of Life Consortium. Validation of the Restless Legs Syndrome Quality of Life Instrument (RLS-QLI): findings of a consortium of national experts and the RLS Foundation. *Qual Life Res*. 2004;13:679-693.

22. Abetz L, Arbuckle R, Allen RP, Mavraki E, Kirsch J. The reliability, validity and responsiveness of the Restless Legs Syndrome Quality of Life questionnaire (RLSQoL) in a trial population. *Health Qual Life Outcomes*. 2005;3:79.

23. Ondo W, Tan EK, Mansoor J. Rheumatologic serologies in secondary restless legs syndrome. *Mov Disord*. 2000;15:321-323.

24. Polydefkis M, Allen RP, Hauer P, Earley CJ, Griffin JW, McArthur JC. Subclinical sensory neuropathy in late-onset restless legs syndrome. *Neurology*. 2000;55:1115-1121.

25. Gemignani F, Brindani F, Negrotti A, Vitetta F, Alfieri S, Marbini A. Restless legs syndrome and polyneuropathy. *Mov Disord*. 2006;21:1254-1257.

26. Gemignani F, Brindani F, Vitetta F, Marbini A, Calzetti S. Restless legs syndrome in diabetic neuropathy: a frequent manifestation of small fiber neuropathy. *J Peripher Nerv Syst*. 2007;12:50-53.

27. Garcia-Borreguero D, Larrosa O, de la Llave Y, Verger K, Masramon X, Hernandez G. Treatment of restless legs syndrome with gabapentin: a double-blind, cross-over study. *Neurology*. 2002;59:1573-1579.

28. Kushida CA, Littner MR, Morgenthaler T, et al. Practice parameters for the indications for polysomnography and related procedures: an update for 2005. *Sleep*. 2005;28:499-521.

6

7

Management

A spectrum of treatment options are available to address the wide range in severity and frequency of restless legs syndrome (RLS) symptoms. This chapter will outline a logical approach for initiating and individualizing treatment for RLS patients.[1] The general guide to treatment decisions is outlined in **Table 7.1**.

Tailoring Treatment to Symptoms

■ When to Treat?

When to treat is a common question that arises with any condition that causes discomfort or pain. When symptoms are frequent and severe, the decision is quite simple: Effective therapy should be instituted promptly. However, this decision is not as straightforward with less severe cases.

Mild and infrequent RLS symptoms often do not need to be treated. However, individuals can differ in their response to symptoms, and even mild and infrequent symptoms may result in significant disability for some.

Decisions on how to treat RLS depend on the degree of discomfort and lifestyle disturbance a particular patient experiences. Most people who experience mild RLS symptoms on an infrequent basis do not need drug therapy. However, if they have problems when sitting for prolonged periods of time, they may not be able to go to the movies or the theater or travel by airplane. Although these symptoms may have no impact on the majority of their life, they may preclude their ability to participate in or enjoy sedentary activities. These restrictions, especially if they impact the ability to work, often require treatment.

TABLE 7.1 — General Guide to Treatment Decisions in Patients With RLS

When to Treat?
- Is RLS clinically significant? Frequent and severe enough to merit treatment?
- If so, what is the appropriate intervention?
  - Consider lifestyle, nonpharmacologic interventions
  - Frequency of symptoms determines when therapy is needed vs daily treatment
  - Severity of symptoms—how bothersome are symptoms? Do they compromise life activities or sleep?

Timing of Doses?
- Time or situation of occurrence of symptoms
- Time to onset of drug action

Adjustment of Treatment
- Routine follow-up
- Monitor for adverse effects, degree of relief
- Be alert to changes in response:
  - Change in patient condition, other treatments, lifestyle changes
  - Consider tolerance, augmentation, and disease progression

Each person with RLS should be assessed for the severity, frequency, and timing of their symptoms. Once these parameters are determined, it should be easier to decide whether to initiate treatment.

It is often difficult to ascertain whether the RLS symptoms are causing enough disruption to warrant treatment. Symptoms are often present for years or even decades before they come to the attention of a physician and are typically downplayed or even ignored. People with RLS tend to believe that the symptoms are normal feelings that everyone may experience or are so strange that they do not deserve to be treated. Once a diagnosis of RLS is made, the patient should be carefully questioned to determine the true degree of suffering and disability from this disorder.

■ Timing of Symptoms

The timing of RLS symptoms is a key factor in the decision of whether and how to treat. Generally, symptoms tend to peak at bedtime but many may experience symptoms earlier or later on in the day. People whose symptoms occur mainly in the early evening or late afternoon have the option of being more active at these times and may not need any drug treatment.

However, if they wish to participate in sedentary activities (movies, theater, travel) at these times, treatment may be essential. With time, most people know which activities and at which times and durations they will provoke their RLS. They can thus take preventive treatment beforehand and completely avoid the emergence of any RLS symptoms.

Symptoms that occur while trying to fall asleep in bed tend to be more troublesome. They can easily disrupt the initiation or maintenance of sleep and result in significant insomnia. However, if the symptoms are mild such that they cause only a short delay in falling asleep, treatment should not be necessary.

Different drugs should be considered depending upon the time that the symptoms occur. Daytime symptoms are better treated with nonsedating drugs, while sedating drugs may be more appropriate for bedtime RLS symptoms. Drugs that onset quickly are better suited for unexpected symptoms (especially at bedtime) while slower-acting drugs can be prescribed for anticipated problems (eg, movies or airplane trips).

■ Frequency and Severity of Symptoms

As previously discussed, mild and infrequent RLS symptoms usually do not need to be treated with medication. These symptoms typically can be managed with nonpharmacologic therapy (see Chapter 8, *Nonpharmacologic Management/Lifestyle Modifications*).

However, RLS symptoms that are very severe but occur infrequently or less-severe RLSL symptoms that occur more frequently may require treatment with drugs. Since it is often hard to determine the severity of RLS symptoms (although several rating scales exist), it may be easier to estimate the severity by the effect the symptoms have on the person's life. Treatment should be considered for any symptoms that are intense enough to be disruptive and affect the person's quality of life.

When symptoms are less severe, treatment may be determined by their frequency. Daily symptoms generally require drug therapy. However, symptoms occurring three to four times per week or more (especially if they cause significant insomnia or disruption of other sedentary activities) may also require daily treatment. It is important to discuss these issues with the patient and determine the impact of their symptoms before prescribing medication.

■ Follow the Patient

Although many patients remain stable for years after starting treatment, it is quite common for RLS to worsen gradually over years to decades. Some patients have wide fluctuations in their symptoms, which may be due to other medications, hormonal changes, concomitant disease, work situation, augmentation (see Chapter 9, *Medications and Other Medical Treatments*), or other reasons that may not always be apparent. It is therefore essential to follow the patient with periodic recheck visits to reassess their symptoms and medication needs.

Medication regimens should be flexible enough to cover the fluctuations that are common among RLS sufferers. Although patients can often prevent RLS symptoms by taking their medication in a timely fashion, this is not always the case. It is a good idea to add a fast-acting medication for those occasions when symptoms present unexpectedly or due to lack of adherence to the medication schedule.

Classification of RLS Patients

There are several ways in which RLS patients may be categorized to help guide treatment protocols. One of the more practical classifications for managing people with RLS was developed by a group of RLS specialists to create an algorithm for guiding the treatment of the disorder.[1] This chapter will discuss this classification, which will be used in subsequent chapters to discuss the management of RLS. It is outlined in **Table 7.2**.

■ Intermittent RLS

Intermittent RLS is defined as RLS that is troublesome enough when present to require treatment but does not occur frequently enough to necessitate daily therapy.[1] These patients are typically easier to manage, as their symptoms tend to be milder and respond more readily to therapy.

Some people with intermittent RLS may experience more intense symptoms, but most in this group

TABLE 7.2 — Classification of RLS Patients
Intermittent RLS Patients • Usually milder • Have significantly bothersome symptoms but not frequent enough to merit daily treatment • Symptoms often situational and/or predictable
Daily RLS Patients • Symptoms frequent enough to merit daily treatment • Usually at least twice a week but usually more frequent and often daily
Refractory RLS Patients • At least one adequate trial of first-line, approved dopamine agonist therapy has failed • Generally indicates that therapeutic effect has diminished; may be due to tolerance, progression, and/or augmentation • Several strategies available for dealing with patient

will complain of these more intense RLS problems only occasionally (airplane flights, long movies, or meetings). With time (often years to decades), it is common for many in this category to progress to more frequent or daily RLS symptoms.

■ Daily RLS

Daily RLS is defined as RLS that is frequent and troublesome enough to require daily therapy.[1] This group tends to have more moderate to severe symptoms. They are also more difficult to treat, often requiring higher doses of medication or even combinations of drugs to relieve their symptoms.

■ Refractory RLS

Refractory RLS is defined as daily RLS treated with a dopamine agonist with one or more of the following outcomes:

- Inadequate initial response despite adequate doses
- Response that has become inadequate with time, despite increasing doses
- Intolerable adverse effects
- Augmentation that is not controllable with additional earlier doses of the drug.

This group tends to be the most difficult to manage. Luckily, they comprise only a small minority of the RLS patients who present to most doctors. Discussion of how to manage and assess these patients is presented in *Chapter 9* and Chapter 10, *Approaching the Patient With RLS*.

REFERENCE

1. Silber MH, Ehrenberg BL, Allen RP, et al; Medical Advisory Board of the Restless Legs Syndrome Foundation. An algorithm for the management of restless legs syndrome. *Mayo Clin Proc*. 2004;79(7):916-922.

8

Nonpharmacologic Management/Lifestyle Modifications

All patients may benefit from the nonpharmacologic management of restless legs syndrome (RLS). **Table 8.1** has a listing of nonpharmacologic approaches and resources. This should be considered for every patient whether they have mild and infrequent symptoms or very severe problems. Many of these interventions will be therapeutic for most people with RLS but others may benefit from only a select few.

Physicians should be familiar with these nonpharmacologic measures since they can provide great relief. Some patients may actually avoid the need for any drugs while others may significantly decrease the amount of medication needed. Therefore, physicians should share this list of nonpharmacologic measures with each patient so that they can discover the ones that may help them. To treat this disorder properly, the doctor and patient must work together as a team, especially with this nondrug approach to the disorder.

Although some of the treatments described in this chapter are either well documented or studied in the medical literature, many others are not. These therapies are often difficult to test in a scientific manner. Therefore, much of the following information is based on anecdotal evidence gathered from those suffering from RLS and experts in the field.

Even though most physicians favor managing RLS with medication, most patients far prefer the nonpharmacologic approach. Whether or not the doctor suggests these therapies, the majority of people with RLS seek them out anyway. Thus it is more beneficial

TABLE 8.1 — Nonpharmacologic Management of RLS

- Avoid provocative substances:
  - Coffee, alcohol, tobacco
  - Medications:
    - Neuroleptics
    - Antidepressants
    - Antihistamines
    - Other dopamine blockers
    - Sedative hypnotics
- Consider RLS-friendly alternatives
- Sleep hygiene:
  - Avoid sleep deprivation
  - Regular hours of sleep
  - Optimize bedroom for sleep
  - Prepare for sleep with relaxing/symptom-reducing activities
- Exercise and physical conditioning
- Alerting activities
- Counterstimulation
- Alternative medical treatments
- Patient organizations and support groups

to work with the patient and guide them to the safer and more effective nondrug treatments.

Avoiding Provocative Substances

As noted, physicians should be familiar with the substances and especially medications that worsen RLS, as these have the potential to become the cause of exacerbating symptoms.

■ Dietary and Nutritional Considerations

Despite the fact that there are few, if any, credible studies investigating the role of diet and nutrition on RLS, this is one of the more common measures employed by people with the disorder and often mentioned in review papers.[1] Those suffering from RLS often report that decreasing carbohydrates or gluten may be helpful. Many report that some dairy products such as ice cream tend to trigger RLS.

There is some literature examining the relationship of caffeine, alcohol, and tobacco and RLS. Although these links have not been firmly established, it is reasonable to suggest that people suffering from RLS abstain from these substances to determine if it improves their symptoms. These substances are further discussed below.

Caffeine

There is an early report[2] in 1978 that discussed 10 patients who had complete relief by withdrawing from caffeine-containing beverages, food, medications, and other xanthine-containing products. Most of the patients got rapid relief from their RLS symptoms within the first few days of abstinence. Two of the patients had a return of symptoms upon the resumption of caffeine products.

One study looking at the risk factors of RLS in depressed or anxious patients maintained on tricyclic and serotonin reuptake inhibiting antidepressants found that the regular use of nonopioid analgesics (frequently combined with caffeine) appeared to be the major risk factor for RLS rather than their use of antidepressants.[3]

Clearly, there is not yet adequate documentation to validate that caffeine exacerbates RLS. Furthermore, as caffeine is an alerting drug, it should decrease the propensity for RLS rather than increase it. Nevertheless, it is prudent to advise people with RLS to determine whether avoiding caffeine is beneficial. This may be difficult due to the pervasiveness of this substance in foods and medications.

Alcohol

Despite alcohol being one of the more commonly used hypnotics, it can cause disturbed sleep. Even a single low dose may result in increased sleep fragmentation and number of awakenings in non–alcohol-dependent adults.[4] Alcohol intake at bedtime shortens the time to onset of sleep but increases wakefulness in the second half of the night,[5] which may then be further exacerbated by the presence of RLS symptoms.

Although no evidence exists to date in the medical literature validating that alcohol exacerbates RLS, this is a common complaint among those with the disorder. It is possible that the sedation created by consuming alcohol may worsen RLS. However, one epidemiologic study using telephone interviews in 1803 Kentucky adults found that RLS was associated with low alcohol consumption.[6]

Tobacco

The association of cigarette smoking and RLS is difficult to discern. An early report describes a 70-year-old female who had been a smoker for 50 years and then stopped due to underlying lung disease.[7] Her RLS symptoms, which had been severe and refractory to all previous therapy, completely disappeared 1 month after smoking cessation.

This relationship of RLS and smoking was not found in an epidemiologic study done in 1997 in 2019 Canadian adults using survey questions asking about RLS symptoms and smoking (people were included as smokers if they smoked in the past 2 weeks).[8] In addition, the investigators studied a group of smokers (at least one cigarette per day) with RLS and periodic limb movements (PLM) and nonsmokers in a sleep laboratory. No significant differences between these groups were found for sleep and motor variables. A major limitation in this study is that the measures of smoking did not take into account nicotine dose, duration of habit, or degree of dependence.

However, an association with smoking (more than one pack per day) was found in the more recent 2000 epidemiologic study noted[6] and a 2004 study that found exsmokers and current smokers were at higher risk for RLS.[9]

■ Considerations for Medications
Neuroleptic Drugs

Neuroleptic drugs, which are used to treat serious psychiatric diseases such as schizophrenia and bipolar disorders, may worsen RLS as they have been found to decrease dopamine neurotransmission.[10] In fact, they are also known to produce akathisia, a condition that shares many clinical features with RLS.[11]

There are case reports in the medical literature that describe the onset of RLS with the following drugs: clozapine,[12] haloperidol,[13] lithium,[14] olanzapine,[15] pimozide,[16] quetiapine,[17] and risperidone.[13] Although there have been no formal studies on these drugs to validate their effect on RLS, many RLS patients have reported worsening symptoms while taking them.

As these medications treat very serious psychiatric conditions, it may be difficult to avoid using them when they are needed. Stopping their use, even when RLS symptoms are clearly exacerbated, should be done with great trepidation due to concerns about worsening the underlying psychiatric disorder. How to manage RLS patients who need this form of therapy is discussed in Chapter 12, *RLS and Psychiatric Disorders*.

Antidepressant Drugs

Similar to the situation with neuroleptic drugs, there are no controlled studies validating the link between antidepressant drugs and worsening RLS symptoms. There are case reports of worsening RLS while on many of the selective serotonin reuptake inhibitors (SSRIs), including citalopram,[18] fluoxetine,[19,20] paroxetine,[21] and sertraline.[22]

Contradicting these reports are two retrospective studies. One reviewed 113 consecutive patients attending a hospital medical clinic who had been prescribed SSRIs (sertraline, paroxetine, or fluoxetine) and found that most patients who had preexisting RLS symptoms (65% of the 113 SSRI patients) experienced improvement of their RLS with their treatment.[23] However, the results of this study may be questioned due to the retrospective design that was unblinded and derived from self-selected questionnaire respondents, which yielded a very high 65% of RLS patients from this SSRI group. A second study reviewed 200 consecutive patients presenting for the evaluation of sleep-initiation insomnia at a sleep-disorders center and did not find any link between antidepressant medication and RLS.[24]

The mechanism of SSRI antidepressant drugs worsening RLS is not fully understood as they do not directly block dopamine. It is thought that the increase in serotonin produced by this class of drugs may exacerbate RLS by serotoninergically mediated inhibition of dopaminergic neurotransmission,[25] which may also explain why they cause akathisia.[26] Additionally, these drugs are known to increase PLM,[27] which are thought to be caused by mechanisms similar to RLS.

Although there are no reported cases of the serotonin-norepinephrine reuptake inhibitors (SNRIs) worsening RLS, patients have complained about duloxetine and venlafaxine exacerbating their RLS. It is thought that the SNRI drugs increase levels of serotonin sufficiently to cause worsening of RLS symptoms. In addition, venlafaxine has been shown to cause as much of an increase in PLM as do the SSRIs.[27]

Mirtazapine, classified as a noradrenergic and specific serotonergic antidepressant, has been linked with worsening RLS. There are several case reports[20,28-32] that describe the exacerbation of RLS with this drug, which may be due to the increased levels of serotonin that it produces.

There are no case reports in the literature about the effect of the tricyclic antidepressants and RLS. However, tricyclic drugs (amitriptyline, clomipramine, doxepin, imipramine, trimipramine) increase levels of serotonin similar to the SSRI medications. Anecdotal reports from patients on tricyclic antidepressants have supported their negative effects on RLS. Additionally, there is one report that describes increased PLM with this class of medication.[33]

Some people have improvement of their RLS symptoms while on antidepressants. This is difficult to explain in light of the many reports of exacerbation of RLS by these drugs. By improving depression and anxiety, these drugs may improve the patient's reaction to their uncomfortable symptoms much like their effect upon the discomfort from neuropathies and musculo-skeletal disorders.

Even when it has been found that an antidepressant is worsening a patient's RLS, the medication may have to be continued, especially when it is being used to treat severe depression or anxiety. *Chapter 12* covers the management of patients with RLS who require these medications.

Antihistamines

Because of their easy availability and widespread use, these drugs are among the most common to worsen RLS. Despite this, there is only one report in the medical literature describing this problem. This study found that diphenhydramine 25 mg, given intravenously, severely exacerbated RLS symptoms.[34] Typically, it is the older, sedating antihistamines that cross the blood-brain barrier that tend to worsen RLS. Many of these are now sold over the counter for control of allergic reactions.

Owing to their ubiquitous presence in combination cold and cough remedies, many people with RLS inadvertently take these drugs and exacerbate their RLS. In addition, people suffering from RLS have trouble falling asleep and will take over-the-counter sleeping pills. These sleep aids generally consist of one of two antihistamines, diphenhydramine or doxylamine, which tend to worsen RLS significantly. RLS patients who take these sleeping pills and do not fall asleep immediately will likely experience increased RLS symptoms that may cause increased insomnia.

Antinausea, Antiemetic, and Antidizzy Medications

Although there are no studies corroborating worsening of RLS with these drugs, there are many patient complaints of this association. Typically, this occurs with the "-zine" drugs (promethazine, hydroxyzine, prochlorperazine, and meclizine). Also included are trimethobenzamide and dimenhydrinate. Most of these drugs are antihistamines or neuroleptics, therefore it is understandable that they may worsen RLS. Additionally, they are all sedating drugs, which may further explain their effect on RLS.

Another antinausea drug, metoclopramide, which is a dopamine receptor antagonist, has been known to exacerbate RLS. Despite this frequent clinical observation, the one medical study that examined this interaction found only a nonsignificant worsening of RLS with metoclopramide.[35]

Sedative Hypnotics

There are many other anecdotal complaints about various other drugs affecting RLS aside from the ones discussed above. However, none has been noted to exacerbate RLS at any significant frequency. There are some concerns with the benzodiazepine class of sedative hypnotics that are often used to treat RLS.

Any medication that induces sedation has a potential to worsen RLS. This was demonstrated in one study that reported moderate worsening of RLS with the intravenous administration of lorazepam.[34] Although these sedatives/anxiolytic drugs may be helpful to promote sleep in RLS sufferers, they should be used with caution during the daytime. Furthermore, the long-acting benzodiazepines may cause daytime drowsiness, which could be counterproductive for treating RLS.

There is one case report of the drug sodium oxybate, which is used for narcolepsy and cataplexy, that was given to a patient with narcolepsy, resulting in a severe new occurrence of typical RLS symptoms that resolved when the drug was discontinued.[36]

■ RLS-Friendly Alternative Drugs

For many of the drugs above that tend to worsen RLS, physicians can prescribe other drugs that do not affect RLS. The more friendly drugs for a number of conditions are listed in **Table 8**.2. The management of RLS in the presence of comorbid psychiatric disorder is covered in *Chapter 12*, and a table listing RLS-friendly drugs for psychiatric treatment is provided in that chapter (**Table 12**.3).

Sleep Hygiene

In review articles, one of the more frequently cited nonpharmacologic treatments for RLS is proper sleep hygiene.[1,37,38] Despite that, there is really no validation of this issue in the medical literature. However, it is thought that getting sufficient sleep to decrease daytime drowsiness should also diminish daytime RLS symptoms.

■ Avoiding Sleep Deprivation

Avoiding sleep deprivation can be a significant problem for those with RLS. As discussed in Chapter

TABLE 8.2 — Alternatives for Dopamine-Blocking Medications for Allergy, Nausea, and Dizziness	
Drugs	**Comments**
Alternatives for Antihistamines	
Loratadine, desloratadine, fexofenadine	These nonsedating drugs do not cross the blood-brain barrier or affect RLS
Steroid, cromolyn, and ipratropium nasal sprays, or montelukast	These are alternatives for treating rhinitis
Alternatives for Antinausea, Antiemetics, Antidizzy Drugs	
Granisetron hydrochloride, ondansetron hydrochloride, dolasetron mesylate	These newer selective 5-hydroxytryptamine receptor antagonists are used to treat the side effects of chemotherapy and do not affect RLS
Transdermal scopolamine patches	This patch is a good alternative to prevent motion sickness and does not worsen RLS
Domperidone	This drug is only available outside the United States. It acts peripherally (does not cross the blood-brain barrier) and does not affect RLS

5, *Consequences*, about 70% of people with moderate to severe RLS take 30 to 60 minutes or longer to fall asleep, and 60% of them experience more than three awakenings per night. Since RLS symptoms occur most often at bedtime, it is easy to see how symptoms interfere with obtaining sufficient sleep.

As many people need to rise at a fixed hour in order to get to work on time, the delay in sleep onset and interrupted sleep cannot be compensated by sleeping later in the morning.

Practicing proper sleep hygiene may be helpful to avoid daytime drowsiness and maintain sufficient alertness to avert an increase in RLS symptoms. The important rules of sleep hygiene that apply to those who suffer from RLS are discussed below.

■ Regular Bedtimes and Rise Times

Standardizing bedtime and wake time can be helpful to strengthen the circadian sleep-wake cycle. This task can be difficult for many RLS sufferers, since their symptoms tend to peak around bedtime. It is common for them to schedule less sedentary activities, such as cleaning the house, in the evening which will permit them to avoid being bothered by RLS symptoms. However, these active endeavors are also more alerting and are not conducive to promoting sleep. If possible, other measures (discussed below) should be implemented that may both relieve the RLS symptoms and promote natural sleepiness.

RLS symptoms follow the body's circadian rhythm, peaking in the evening/bedtime and waning throughout the sleep period until its nadir at about 10 AM.[39,40] Therefore, many people who experience bothersome RLS symptoms at night will be forced to delay their bedtime for several hours until their symptoms begin to naturally wane. Generally, the more severe the RLS, the longer it takes for the nighttime symptoms to wane sufficiently to allow sleep. Many may not be able to fall asleep before 3 AM to 6 AM, which can make it difficult to get up a few hours later for work.

Shift work usually presents challenges for patients with insomnia, who do poorly with variable bedtimes and wake times, and it may be even harder for those with insomnia induced by RLS. It may seem that the evening or night shift would be helpful for those with RLS since they could be active when symptoms tend to be maximal. This schedule may work for a few days but as the circadian rhythm resets (as this rhythm is more dependent upon the wake time), the RLS symptoms will also shift back to bedtime. The same is true for people who do not have to get up at a fixed time to work and start going to bed later and sleeping later. Within several days, they will have simply shifted their circadian cycles and RLS problems to a different time of day.

As discussed, regular rise times are important to maintain proper function of the circadian rhythm. Even if people have the option of sleeping in, it is recommended that they get out of bed at the same time each day. This aspect of sleep is much easier to accomplish by simply using an alarm clock. Due to social and other pressures, it is usually more difficult to maintain a regular bedtime, especially when also being plagued by RLS symptoms that force one out of bed.

■ Prepare the Bedroom

Having a bedroom environment that is conducive to falling asleep is important for people with insomnia and even more so for those with RLS. Thus people with RLS should follow some of the general measures recommended for those with insomnia.

This includes controlling the temperature as well as the noise and light levels. Temperature is an individual preference and can be set accordingly. Loud snoring from bed partners, sounds of people talking, or television and traffic noises can disrupt sleep. Although these disturbances cannot always be avoided, people can employ measures to reduce their effects. White noise generators (eg, the SoundScreen or CD players with sounds of rain, waves, wind, etc) can obscure most moderate level noises. Depending upon the time of year and location, the intrusion of daylight may interrupt sleep. Blinds, blackout curtains, or other means are recommended to keep the room dark.

The bed itself can be important. Movements by bed partners can easily disturb sleep. Most people with insomnia toss and turn frequently, and this is an even bigger problem for those with RLS. Due to the urge to move their legs, they usually need more room and are anxious about disturbing their bed partner. A solution to this problem is to either get twin beds (that can be separated by ½ inch at sleep time) or a king-size bed made of viscoelastic foam (such as a TempurPedic) that diminishes any movement. Bed covers and blankets can be an issue for many with RLS. Some prefer tight or heavy covers, while others cannot have any contact with their blanket.

With all of these issues that may not always have an easy alternative (ie, a bed partner snoring very loudly), it is often beneficial to have an alternate bedroom in which to sleep. Additionally, RLS sufferers may feel that they need to be completely free to move and calm their restless legs without worrying about the effect on their bed partner. It is not unusual for them to have strange sleep positions that soothe their legs enough to enable them to sleep. This includes having their feet propped up on the back of a couch or sleeping on the floor with their legs propped up against the wall.

■ Presleep Activity

One of the recommendations for sleep hygiene is to establish a prebedtime routine that helps one unwind. This is much easier for most people with insomnia, but those with RLS usually cannot perform the sedentary activities that are relaxing while their symptoms are peaking before bedtime. In fact, relaxing may be counterproductive.

Many people with RLS choose counterstimulation techniques (see below) or other activities that calm their RLS. One of the more common counterstimulation techniques includes taking hot baths or showers. Some prefer cold water while others may alternate hot and cold water (using the bathtub faucet), running the water over their legs for 5 to 15 minutes. Alternatively, hot or cold packs are sometimes used. This may provide a few minutes of relief, often enough to help the sleep-deprived person fall asleep.

Other common counterstimulation practices involve rubbing the legs, massages, stretches, deep knee bends, and other activities that work the leg muscles. The duration needed to get relief can vary considerably.

Exercise

Moderate-intensity exercise has been recommended for people with insomnia as it has been shown to increase slow wave (stages 3 and 4 deep) sleep,[41] sleep duration,[42] and sleep efficiencies,[43,44] and to decrease awakenings[45] and decrease the latency to sleep onset.[46] Additionally, the timing of exercise may be important in that some studies have demonstrated that these benefits accrue only with morning exercise but not with evening exercise.[46,47] These suggestions can also be applied to those with RLS, except as noted, when their preference for evening exercise may be counterproductive.

Exercise may have other direct benefits for RLS sufferers. One study found that people with RLS showed improvement with a 12-week conditioning program of aerobic and lower-body resistance training 3 days per week when compared with those who did not exercise.[45] However, this benefit seems to occur only with moderate exercise; it is common for vigorous exercise (running, training for competition, etc) to markedly worsen RLS symptoms. This may occur even when exercising too energetically in the morning and the negative effects may last for several days.

Therefore, the best advice for patients with RLS is to exercise regularly at moderate intensity early in the day. Prebedtime exercise or stretching routines should be as short as possible to avoid increasing alertness and thus promoting insomnia.

Mental Alerting Activities

RLS symptoms tend to occur with physical or mental inactivity. Therefore, activities that promote alertness (which in turn activates the body's motor systems) may be particularly helpful to abate RLS symptoms, especially when physical movement is otherwise restricted. Situations such as travel (especially by airplane when the fasten-seat-belt sign is on), meetings, or religious services are typical examples that benefit from alerting measures.

Almost any activity that requires thinking will relieve RLS symptoms. Below is a list of common activities that help RLS:
- Playing cards, such as solitaire if alone
- Playing computer or video games
- Knitting, needlework, or other handwork
- Working on a crossword or other puzzles
- Engaging in an interesting discussion or argument
- Balancing a checkbook, homework, paperwork, or working with spreadsheets
- Writing a diary, letter, or internet blog
- Listening to music actively
- Reading an engrossing book.

As long as the person engages in these activities, the RLS symptoms will be controlled. Often, keeping mentally alert can relieve symptoms for hours, which is long enough for most domestic airplane trips.

Counterstimulation Techniques

These techniques have already been discussed somewhat in other sections, as they are useful for coping with many situations that cause RLS symptoms, especially when medication is not effective or available. It is thought that these counterstimulation procedures work much the same way that shaking one's hand helps abate the pain from hitting a finger with a hammer.

Most of these activities are focused on the legs but also apply to other affected body parts, such as the arms:

- Hot or cold baths or showers
- Run hot or cold water on the legs (or alternate the temperatures every few minutes)
- Cold or hot packs applied to the legs
- Electric blankets
- Leg massage (manual or electrical)
- Leg tickling
- Leg wraps (eg, Ace bandages), surgical support stockings
- Sexual activity and orgasm (although in some cases this may worsen RLS).

The duration that these techniques need to be done can be quite variable. Often a few minutes can provide long enough relief so that the RLS sufferer can go to bed and fall asleep before symptoms return and cause insomnia.

Alternative Treatments

Despite the general lack of medical evidence, many people who are frustrated with the traditional/pharmacologic treatments for RLS or other chronic conditions turn to alternative therapies. There is a broad range of remedies from which to choose. Despite their lack of proven efficacy or recommendations from traditional doctors, a large percentage of patients will seek them out. Physicians should be aware of these treatments, as patients wish to discuss them or are already using them.

■ Complimentary and Alternative Medicine (CAM)

These therapies are divided into five main categories. Few scientific medical studies have examined any of these treatments for relief of RLS. However, due to the overwhelming interest and use of CAM, the National Institutes of Health has established the National Center for Complementary and Alternative Medicine (NCCAM). Its website (*www.nccam.nih.gov*) is informative and an excellent resource for research, education, training, and news on CAM.

Alternative Medical Systems

These are separate medical systems that are built upon complete systems of theory and practice, which differ from conventional medicine. Examples include homeopathic medicine, naturopathic medicine, traditional Chinese medicine, and ayurveda (East Indian therapy based on diet and herbal remedies that emphasizes the use of body, mind, and spirit in disease prevention and treatment).

Acupuncture and acupressure are among the more common of these modalities that people seek for disorders that cause pain or discomfort. Only two articles have been published so far, both in the Chinese traditional medicine literature.[48] Whether this therapy is effective outside of China remains to be determined but so far, sporadic anecdotal reports from RLS sufferers have not been very positive.

Mind-Body Interventions

This category involves techniques designed to enhance the mind's capacity to affect bodily functions and symptoms. Examples include meditation, prayer, mental healing, and therapies that use creative outlets such as art, music, or dance.

Biologically Based Therapies

These therapies use substances found in nature, such as herbs, foods, and vitamins. These are among the most popular treatments used by RLS patients and are readily purchased from health food stores, pharmacies, and on the internet.

Manipulative and Body-Based Methods

These methods are based on manipulation and/or movement of one or more parts of the body. Some examples include chiropractic or osteopathic manipulation and massage.

Energy Therapies

Biofield therapies (energy fields that purportedly surround and penetrate the human body but have never been scientifically proved) and bioelectromagnetic-based therapies (unconventional use of electromagnetic fields, such as pulsed fields, magnetic fields, or alternating-current or direct-current fields) make up this category.

■ Chiropractic Medicine

People see chiropractors for many different ailments including pain. Currently, there are no medical studies or reports on this modality for treating RLS. Sporadic anecdotal reports so far do not indicate that this treatment is helpful for RLS symptoms.

Patient Organizations and Support Groups

Many patients with RLS feel isolated as if they are the only ones with the disorder. This belief is changing somewhat due to the increased awareness that RLS has received over the past few years, but it is still all too common. Joining a patient organization or support group is one of the best ways to combat the problem of isolation and at the same time become educated about the disorder.

The RLS Foundation (*www.rls.org*) is an international nonprofit RLS organization based in Rochester, Minnesota, that has advocated for and helped RLS patients since its inception in 1992. Their website contains information for patients on every aspect of RLS, including a list of doctors who treat RLS. Brochures can be obtained on many RLS topics and they publish a quarterly newsletter, *NightWalkers*. They also supply a medical alert card that details the drugs that patients should avoid.

A more complete discussion of the RLS foundation resources and activities and a list of other patient support resources can be found in Appendix B.

REFERENCES

1. Stiasny K, Oertel W Hm Trenkwalder C. Clinical symptomatology and treatment of restless legs syndrome and periodic limb movement disorder. *Sleep Med Rev.* 2002;6:253-265.
2. Lutz EG. Restless legs, anxiety and caffeinism. *J Clin Psychiatry.* 1978;39:693-698.
3. Leutgeb U, Martus P. Regular intake of non-opioid analgesics is associated with an increased risk of restless legs syndrome in patients maintained on antidepressants. *Eur J Med Res.* 2002;7:368-378.
4. Rouhani S, Tran G, Leplaideur F, Durlach J, Poenaru S. EEG effects of a single low dose of ethanol on afternoon sleep in the nonalcohol-dependent adult. *Alcohol.* 1989;6:687-690.

5. Roth T, Roehrs T, Zorick F, Conway W. Pharmacological effects of sedative-hypnotics, narcotic analgesics, and alcohol during sleep. *Med Clin North Am*. 1985;69:1281-1288.

6. Phillips B, Young T, Finn L, Asher K, Hening WA, Purvis C. Epidemiology of restless legs symptoms in adults. *Arch Intern Med*. 2000;160:2137-2141.

7. Mountifield JA. Restless leg syndrome relieved by cessation of smoking. *CMAJ*. 1985;133:426-427.

8. Lavigne GL, Lobbezoo F, Rompre PH, Nielsen TA, Montplaisir J. Cigarette smoking as a risk factor or an exacerbating factor for restless legs syndrome and sleep bruxism. *Sleep*. 1997;20:290-293.

9. Berger K, Luedemann J, Trenkwalder C, John U, Kessler C. Sex and the risk of restless legs syndrome in the general population. *Arch Intern Med*. 2004;164:196-202.

10. Chiodo LA. Dopamine-containing neurons in the mammalian central nervous system: electrophysiology and pharmacology. *Neurosci Biobehav Rev*. 1988;12:49-91.

11. Walters AS, Hening W, Rubinstein M, Chokroverty S. A clinical and polysomnographic comparison of neuroleptic-induced akathisia and the idiopathic restless legs syndrome. *Sleep*. 1991;14:339-345.

12. Duggal HS, Mendhekar DN. Clozapine-associated restless legs syndrome. *J Clin Psychopharmacol*. 2007;27:89-90.

13. Wetter TC, Brunner J, Bronisch T. Restless legs syndrome probably induced by risperidone treatment. *Pharmacopsychiatry*. 2002;35:109-111.

14. Terao T, Terao M, Yoshimura R, Abe K. Restless legs syndrome induced by lithium. *Biol Psychiatry*. 1991;30:1167-1170.

15. Kraus T, Schuld A, Pollmacher T. Periodic leg movements in sleep and restless legs syndrome probably caused by olanzapine. *J Clin Psychopharmacol*. 1999;19:478-479.

16. Montplaisir J, Lorrain D, Godbout R. Restless legs syndrome and periodic leg movements in sleep: the primary role of dopaminergic mechanism. *Eur Neurol*. 1991;31:41-43.

17. Pinninti NR, Mago R, Townsend J, Doghramji K. Periodic restless legs syndrome associated with quetiapine use: a case report. *J Clin Psychopharmacol*. 2005;25:617-618.

18. Perroud N, Lazignac C, Baleydier B, Cicotti A, Maris S, Damsa C. Restless legs syndrome induced by citalopram: a psychiatric emergency? *Gen Hosp Psychiatry*. 2007;29:72-74.

19. Bakshi R. Fluoxetine and restless legs syndrome. *J Neurol Sci*. 1996;142:151-152.

20. Prospero-Garcia KA, Torres-Ruiz A, Ramirez-Bermudez J, Velazquez-Moctezuma J, Arana-Lechuga Y, Teran-Perez G. Fluoxetine-mirtazapine interaction may induce restless legs syndrome: report of 3 cases from a clinical trial. *J Clin Psychiatry*. 2006;67:1820.

136

21. Sanz-Fuentenebro FJ, Huidobro A, Tejadas-Rivas A. Restless legs syndrome and paroxetine. *Acta Psychiatr Scand*. 1996;94(6):482-484.

22. Hargrave R, Beckley DJ. Restless leg syndrome exacerbated by sertraline. *Psychosomatics*. 1998;39:177-178.

23. Dimmitt SB, Riley GJ. Selective serotonin receptor uptake inhibitors can reduce restless legs symptoms. *Arch Intern Med*. 2000;160:712.

24. Brown LK, Dedrick DL, Doggett JW, Guido PS. Antidepressant medication use and restless legs syndrome in patients presenting with insomnia. *Sleep Med*. 2005;6:443-450.

25. Lipinski JF Jr, Mallya G, Zimmerman P, Pope HG Jr. Fluoxetine-induced akathisia: clinical and theoretical implications. *J Clin Psychiatry*. 1989;50:339-342.

26. Baldassano CF, Truman CJ, Nierenberg A, Ghaemi SN, Sachs GS. Akathisia: a review and case report following paroxetine treatment. *Compr Psychiatry*. 1996;37:122-124.

27. Yang C, White DP, Winkelman JW. Antidepressants and periodic leg movements of sleep. *Biol Psychiatry*. 2005;58:510-514.

28. Bonin B, Vandel P, Kantelip JP. Mirtazapine and restless leg syndrome: a case report. *Therapie*. 2000;55:655-656.

29. Bahk WM, Pae CU, Chae JH, Jun TY, Kim KS. Mirtazapine may have the propensity for developing a restless legs syndrome? A case report. *Psychiatry Clin Neurosci*. 2002;56:209-210.

30. Teive HA, de Quadros A, Barros FC, Werneck LC. Worsening of autosomal dominant restless legs syndrome after use of mirtazapine: case report. *Arq Neuropsiquiatr*. 2002;60:1025-1029.

31. Agargun MY, Kara H, Ozbek H, Tombul T, Ozer OA. Restless legs syndrome induced by mirtazapine. *J Clin Psychiatry*. 2002;63:1179.

32. Pae CU, Kim TS, Kim JJ, et al. Re-administration of mirtazapine could overcome previous mirtazapine- associated restless legs syndrome? *Psychiatry Clin Neurosci*. 2004;58:669-670.

33. Garvey MJ, Tollefson GD. Occurrence of myoclonus in patients treated with cyclic antidepressants. *Arch Gen Psychiatry*. 1987;44:269-272.

34. Allen RP, Lesage S, Earley CJ. Anti-histamines and benzodiazepines exacerbate daytime restless legs syndrome (RLS) symptoms. *Sleep*. 2005;28:A279. Abstract.

35. Winkelmann J, Schadrack J, Wetter TC, Zieglgansberger W, Trenkwalder C. Opioid and dopamine antagonist drug challenges in untreated restless legs syndrome patients. *Sleep Med*. 2001;2:57-61.

36. Abril B, Carlander B, Touchon J, Dauvilliers Y. Restless legs syndrome in narcolepsy: a side effect of sodium oxybate? *Sleep Med.* 2007;8:181-183.

37. Paulson GW. Restless legs syndrome. How to provide symptom relief with drug and nondrug therapies. *Geriatrics.* 2000;55:35-38.

38. Hening W, Allen R, Earley C, Kushida C, Picchietti D, Silber M. The treatment of restless legs syndrome and periodic limb movement disorder. An American Academy of Sleep Medicine Review. *Sleep.* 1999;22:970-999.

39. Trenkwalder C, Hening WA, Walters AS, Campbell SS, Rahman K, Chokroverty S. Circadian rhythm of periodic limb movements and sensory symptoms of restless legs syndrome. *Mov Disord.* 1999;14:102-110.

40. Hening WA, Walters AS, Wagner M, et al. Circadian rhythm of motor restlessness and sensory symptoms in the idiopathic restless legs syndrome. *Sleep.* 1999;22:901-912

41. Naylor E, Penev PD, Orbeta L, et al. Daily social and physical activity increases slow-wave sleep and daytime neuropsychological performance in the elderly. *Sleep.* 2000;23:87-95.

42. King AC, Oman RF, Brassington GS, Bliwise DL, Haskell WL. Moderate-intensity exercise and self-rated quality of sleep in older adults. A randomized controlled trial. *JAMA.* 1997;277:32-37.

43. Norman JF, Von Essen SG, Fuchs RH, McElligott M. Exercise training effect on obstructive sleep apnea syndrome. *Sleep Res Online.* 2000;3:121-129.

44. Shapiro CM, Warren PM, Trinder J, et al. Fitness facilitates sleep. *Eur J Appl Physiol Occup Physiol.* 1984;53:1-4.

45. Aukerman MM, Aukerman D, Bayard M, Tudiver F, Thorp L, Bailey B. Exercise and restless legs syndrome: a randomized controlled trial. *J Am Board Fam Med.* 2006;19:487-493.

46. Youngstedt SD, O'Connor PJ, Dishman RK. The effects of acute exercise on sleep: a quantitative synthesis. *Sleep.* 1997;20:203-214.

47. Tworoger SS, Yasui Y, Vitiello MV, et al. Effects of a yearlong moderate-intensity exercise and a stretching intervention on sleep quality in postmenopausal women. *Sleep.* 2003;26:830-836.

48. Hu J. Acupuncture treatment of restless leg syndrome. *J Tradit Chin Med.* 2001;21:312-316.

9

Medications and Other Medical Treatments

When nonpharmacologic therapy is no longer adequate, treatment with drugs should be strongly considered (as discussed in Chapter 7, *Management*). The recent approval of two dopamine agonists—pramipexole and ropinirole—in the United States and Europe has made the starting point for treatment clearer. But there are many other effective drugs that have been studied for restless legs syndrome (RLS) and we have tried to indicate how they, too, may be used and what their advantages and disadvantages might be. In general, RLS experts have become familiar with four classes of drugs that are most useful in treating RLS (**Table 9**.1):

- Dopaminergics
- Anticonvulsants
- Opioids
- Sedative hypnotics.

Dopaminergic Medications

The first dopaminergic medication used in RLS was L-dopa. L-dopa is a precursor drug in that it is enzymatically modified by dopa decarboxylase into the active neurotransmitter, dopamine. An L-dopa containing drug was the first dopaminergic used to treat RLS in modern times by Sevket Akpinar, a Turkish neurologist, in 1982.[1] When RLS patients started taking L-dopa, it was as if their troublesome symptoms were magically relieved. However, after an initial dramatic period of relief, the majority who took these drugs on a daily basis began experiencing a marked worsening of their

TABLE 9.1 — Drug Classes Used in RLS
Dopaminergics 　• Levodopa combined with a decarboxylase inhibition 　• Dopamine agonists: 　　– Ropinirole 　　– Pramipexole
Anticonvulsants 　• Gabapentin and related drugs 　• Others
Opioids 　• Mild, moderate, and strong for different situations
Sedative hypnotics 　• Benzodiazepines 　• Nonbenzodiazepines

RLS symptoms (called augmentation, see below).[2] Due to this problem of augmentation, it is recommended that L-dopa should not be used on a daily basis unless it is effective at a very low dose (<200 mg/day). As a consequence, over the past decade, the dopamine agonists have now become the favored medications for daily treatment. This has led to the registration of dopamine agonists for RLS. Ropinirole (May, 2005) and pramipexole (November, 2006) were the first to be approved in the United States with the reverse order in Europe. All dopaminergic drugs have been at least temporarily effective in RLS and all share a spectrum of adverse effects. These are detailed in **Table 9.2**. Individual drugs may be more or less associated with specific side effects, as discussed below.

Dopamine Agonists

Dopamine agonists are the drugs of choice for daily RLS symptoms.[3] They are the only drugs that have been approved for treatment of idiopathic RLS in both Europe and the United States. Therefore, physi-

TABLE 9.2 — Dopaminergic Side Effects

Common Acute Adverse Effects
- Nausea; less commonly, vomiting
- Light headedness; rarely, syncope
- Headache
- Somnolence
- Insomnia

Less Common Adverse Effects
- Peripheral edema
- Sleep attacks
- Impulse control disorders:
  – Hypersexuality
  – Pathologic gambling
  – Excessive shopping

Subacute to Late Onset Adverse Effects
- Augmentation:
  – Advance in time of onset of symptoms
  – Greater severity of symptoms when present
  – Reduced latency to onset of symptoms at rest
  – Spread of symptoms to involve new body parts

Adverse Effects Primarily Shown in Parkinson's Disease
- Dyskinesias
- Hallucinations
- Psychosis

Adverse Effects Associated With Ergoline Derivatives
- Fibrotic syndromes
  – Retroperitoneal fibrosis
  – Pleuropulmonary fibrosis
  – Fibrotic cardiomyopathy

Adverse Effects Associated With Transdermal Dopaminergics
- Application site reaction

cians should become familiar with these drugs and be comfortable using them to treat RLS. Currently, two dopamine agonists (pramipexole and ropinirole) are approved for treating RLS. **Table 9.3** lists the dopamine agonists and their usual doses.

TABLE 9.3 — Dopamine Agonists

Generic Drug Name	Half-Life in Hours	Route Metabolized or Eliminated	Ergot Alkaloid Derivative	Doses per Day	Individual Dose Range (mg)	Average Daily Dose (mg)	Approved for Treating RLS
Apomorphine (subcutaneous)	½-1	Unknown	No	1-?	?	?	No
Bromocriptine	3-12	Liver	Yes	1-3	2.5-10	10-15	No
Cabergoline	>65	Liver	Yes	1	0.25-4	1.5-2	No
Lisuride	2-3	Liver	Yes	1	0.1-0.4	0.3	No
Pergolide	7-16	Liver	Yes	1-3	0.05-1.0	0.25-0.5	No
Piribedil (sustained release)	21	?	No	1	25-350	50-150	No
Pramipexole	8-12	Kidney	No	1-3	0.125-1.5	0.25-0.5	Yes
Ropinirole	6	Liver	No	1-3	0.25-4	0.5-2	Yes
Rotigotine (transdermal)	3 initial, 5-7 terminal	Liver, then excreted by the kidneys	No	1	1-3	1-3	No
Terguride	4	Kidney	Yes	1-3	0.25-0.75	0.5	No

■ **Approved Medications** *(in alphabetical order)*
  Pramipexole

Pramipexole was the second drug approved by the Food and Drug Administration (FDA) for the treatment of moderate-to-severe primary RLS in the United States. Similar to ropinirole, many studies have confirmed its efficacy in RLS.[4-9]

Two large (n=344 or 345) double-blinded, placebo-controlled trials evaluated efficacy and safety of pramipexole treatment of primary RLS with a randomization giving twice as many subjects on pramipexole as placebo. The primary end points in both studies were the clinical global improvement and the change from baseline in IRLS. The European study[9] with individually titrated doses ranging from 0.125 or 0.75 (median pramipexole dose of 0.35 mg/day) reported response after 6 weeks of treatment. The mean IRLS-score decreases were 5.7 for placebo and 12.3 for pramipexole. The percentage much/very much improved was 32.5% on placebo and 62.9% on pramipexole (**Figure 9.1**).

In the second study conducted in the United States,[7] patients were randomized to placebo or one of three fixed pramipexole doses: 0.25, 0.5, or 0.75 mg/day. Responses at 12 weeks showed decreases on the IRLS of 9.3 for placebo vs 12.8 for 0.25 mg pramipexole, 13.8 for 0.5 mg, and 14.1 for 0.75 mg (**Figure 9.1**). The percentage much/very much improved on the CGI was 51.2% for placebo vs 74.7% for 0.25 pramipexole, 67.9% for 0.5 mg, and 72.9% for 0.75 mg. In addition, 150 RLS patients who had responded to pramipexole were then randomly switched to either placebo or continuing on their pramipexole and followed for another 3 months.[6] The percentage of patients with predcfined worsening of their RLS scale and also a decrease in CGI was 85.5% for placebo and 20.5% for pramipexole treatment.

A third study was a dose-finding parallel-group polysomnography study in which a total of 109 patients

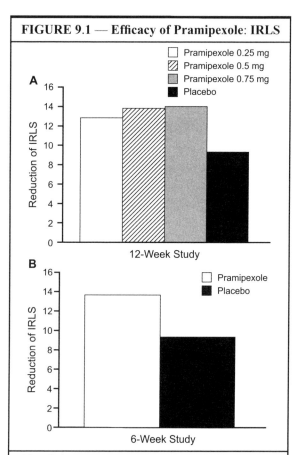

FIGURE 9.1 — Efficacy of Pramipexole: IRLS

Abbreviation: IRLS, International Restless Legs Syndrome Rating Scale.

A) This was a 12-week fixed-dose trial of pramipexole in comparison with placebo.[1] There was a significant reduction of the IRLS summed score at each dose level. *B)* This was a 6-week flexible-dose study of pramipexole compared with placebo.[2] There was a significant reduction of the IRLS summed score; mean pramipexole dose at measurement was 0.35 mg/day.

[1]Winkelman JW, et al. *Neurology*. 2006;67:1034-1039; [2]Oertel WH, et al. *Mov Disord*. 2007;22:213-219.

were randomly administered one of the following: placebo, 0.125 mg, 0.25 mg, 0.5 mg, or 0.75 mg for 3 weeks.[5] The PLMI was reduced in all four drug groups by about 80% compared with placebo (**Figure 9.2**). The IRLS score was lower for all drug doses compared with placebo, with the higher doses showing >50% reduction.[5] In summary, these three larger trials showed that pramipexole is efficacious in RLS at doses ranging from 0.25 to 0.75 mg per day (**Figure 9.1**). These studies also provided evidence that pramipexole improved sleep and quality of life in RLS patients.

As noted in **Table 9.3**, pramipexole has a half-life of 8 to 12 hours (young-older subjects) and is excreted through the kidneys. Drugs that are inhibitors of renal

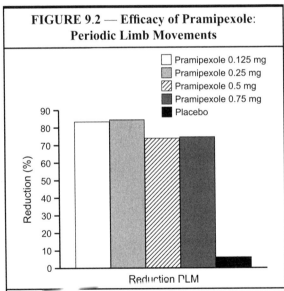

FIGURE 9.2 — Efficacy of Pramipexole: Periodic Limb Movements

Legend:
- ☐ Pramipexole 0.125 mg
- ▨ Pramipexole 0.25 mg
- ▨ Pramipexole 0.5 mg
- ▨ Pramipexole 0.75 mg
- ■ Placebo

Reduction (%) vs Reduction PLM

This study was a 3-week fixed-dose study using pramipexole doses from 0.125 to 0.75 mg compared with placebo. Reduction of periodic limb movement index, both awake and asleep, was significant at each dose level.

Partinen M, et al. *Sleep Med.* 2006;7:407-417.

tubular secretion of organic bases via the cationic transport system (eg, cimetidine, ranitidine, diltiazem, triamterene, verapamil, quinidine, and quinine) decrease the elimination of pramipexole.

Pramipexole is approved for use in moderate to severe primary RLS once daily at 2 to 3 hours before bedtime. It has been used off label up to three times daily (2 to 3 hours before the onset of symptoms) for patients with symptoms that occur substantially before bedtime. Its onset of effective action is a little slower than that of ropinirole, taking 2 to 3 hours to reach optimal effect. Like ropinirole, it is fully absorbed with food, but will then have a 1-hour delay in its onset of action.

Typically, the drug should be started at 0.125 mg then titrated to effect. In the United States, the starter pack increases to 0.25 mg after 5 days. Dose may be increased to 0.5 mg in another 4 to 7 days if necessary. Some specialists titrate as slow as incrementing by 0.125 mg weekly, although some others proceed more rapidly. More gradual titration schedules tend to limit side effects. Most patients respond to doses of 0.25 mg to 0.5 mg, while doses above 0.75 mg are reserved for use off-label in those with very severe RLS.

Adverse reactions are similar to the dopamine effects listed in **Table 9**.**2**.

Ropinirole

Ropinirole was the first dopamine agonist approved in the United States (May 2005) by the FDA for treating moderate-to-severe primary RLS. It was later approved in Europe. Several studies have confirmed the efficacy of this drug in RLS.[10-13] The three major trials followed similar methodology. Each trial lasted 12 weeks, with the dose of ropinirole being titrated upward in an unforced paradigm from 0.25 mg to a maximum of 4 mg administered in a single dose 1 to 3 hours before bed. The primary end point was the IRLS in two studies[10,11] and the PLMI on PSG in the third.[12]

The mean dose used in the three studies was 1.8 or 1.9 mg. The IRLS scores were significantly lower with ropinirole compared with placebo. The degree of difference between the placebo and treatment groups was 3.0[10] and 2.5.[11] In the third study, ropinirole resulted in a significant 70% decrease in PLMS and 61% decrease in PLMW compared with placebo.[12] In summary, ropinirole provided both subjective benefit to patients with RLS (**Figure 9**.3) and reduced their involuntary movements (PLM) at night (**Figure 9**.4). Additional measures of sleep and quality of life also showed greater benefit with ropinirole than with placebo in these studies.

As noted in **Table 9.3**, this drug has a half-life of 6 hours and is metabolized in the liver. Ropinirole does not affect the metabolism of other drugs but its metabolism is slowed by inhibitors of CYP1A2, such as ciprofloxacin, and by estrogens.

Ropinirole is approved for use in moderate to severe primary RLS with once-daily dosing to treat bedtime symptoms. As the drug may take 1 to 3 hours to exert its clinical effects, it should be taken 1 to 3 hours before bedtime. However, some people may benefit from its effects in as fast as 30 minutes.

Ropinirole should be started at its lowest dose of 0.25 mg and then titrated slowly as necessary. In the United States, a starter kit increases the dose to 0.5 mg after 2 days of 0.25 mg, then to 1 mg daily after 1 week. If higher doses are needed, the dose may be incremented by 0.5 mg on a weekly basis to a 3 mg and, in the seventh week, by 1 mg to the maximum of 4 mg. Most patients do well with lower doses of between 0.5 to 2 mg per day. Some specialists prefer more gradual titration schedules, incrementing the dose by 0.25 mg or 0.5 mg every 5 to 7 days as this may decrease the frequency and intensity of side effects.

Despite its once-daily indication, ropinirole has been used off label by experts in split doses to treat

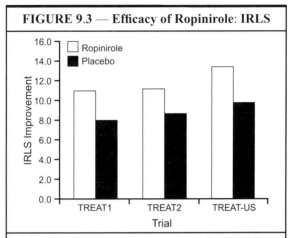

FIGURE 9.3 — Efficacy of Ropinirole: IRLS

Abbreviations: IRLS, International Restless Legs Syndrome Rating Scale; TREAT, Therapy with Ropinirole; Efficacy and Tolerability.

The reduction in the IRLS is given for ropinirole and placebo in three flexible dose studies: TREAT1,[1] TREAT2,[2] and TREAT-US.[3] All studies lasted 12 weeks. Mean doses at the time of measurements were: 1.9, 1.5, and 2.1 mg/day, respectively. Each trial showed a significant reduction of the IRLS score in the ropinirole group compared with placebo.

[1]Trenkwalder C, et al. *J Neurol Neurosurg Psychiatry*. 2004; 75:92-97; [2]Walters AS, et al. *Mov Disord*. 2004;19:1414-1423; [3]Bogan RK, et al. *Mayo Clin Proc*. 2006;81:17-27.

symptoms that occur earlier in the day. Typically, this drug was prescribed 1 to 3 hours before the onset of symptoms up to three times daily, with the first dose given upon awakening, if necessary.

Adverse Dopamine Side Effects

Adverse effects of pramipexole and ropinirole, and the dopaminergic drugs generally, are outlined in **Table 9.2**. Most of these adverse effects are common to all dopamine drugs. The most common side effect is

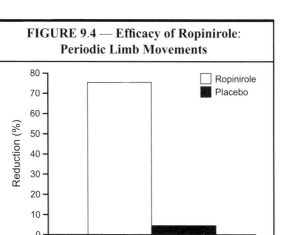

FIGURE 9.4 — Efficacy of Ropinirole: Periodic Limb Movements

The reduction in the periodic limb movement index in a 12-week flexible-dose comparison of ropinirole to placebo. Mean dose of ropinirole at the end of the study was 1.8 mg.

Allen R, et al. *Sleep*. 2004;27:907-914.

nausea that tends to occur with initiating these drugs or with increasing their dose. Generally, the nausea lasts only several hours after a dose and may cease after a few days on a stable dose. Taking the medication with food often mitigates the nausea but delays the onset of action by about 1 hour. Other common adverse reactions include somnolence, vomiting, dizziness, fatigue, postural hypotension, and insomnia. Some people have to discontinue the medication due to these problems but most can maintain treatment, as the reactions are often transient and mild.

The package insert warns about an increased risk of melanoma. However, this is due to the increased incidence of melanoma with Parkinson's disease, even though no dopamine agonist has yet been linked to melanoma. Occasional reports of hallucinations have also been noted with these drugs during RLS treatment, but these are much more common with the higher doses used for Parkinson's disease.

Compulsive behavior (gambling, hypersexuality, eating, etc) is a new treatment-emergent problem that occurs rarely in those with RLS[14,15] compared with patients with Parkinson's disease.[16-18] This problem appears to be a dose-dependant phenomenon (decreasing the dose often resolves the issue), which may explain the increased incidence in the Parkinson's disease patients who use much higher doses.

There have been warnings about sudden sleep attacks, but this problem is also more of a concern with the higher doses used for Parkinson's disease. Doctors should apprise patients of all of these potential risks but should put them in proper perspective.

Rebound and augmentation are two problems of extended treatment. The features of these are given in **Table 9.4** and discussed below after the section on L-dopa.

■ L-Dopa
Varied Formulations

There are two currently available forms of L-dopa: combined with carbidopa in the United States (approved only for treating Parkinson's disease and not for RLS) and combined with benserazide outside the United States (approved in Europe for the treatment of RLS). Carbidopa and benserazide act only outside the central nervous system (CNS) to inhibit the enzyme dopa decarboxylase from converting L-dopa into dopamine, thus decreasing the peripheral side effects and increasing the amount of L-dopa available in the brain, which reduces the required dose.

The immediate-release formulations of L-dopa may have an onset as quickly as 15 to 30 minutes on an empty stomach, which makes them useful for unexpected episodes of RLS that need rapid relief. However, these immediate-release drugs have a very

TABLE 9.4 — Max Planck Institute Diagnostic Criteria for Augmentation*

A. Basic features *(all of which need to be met)*:
- The increase in symptom severity experienced on 5 out of 7 days during the previous week
- The increase in symptom severity not accounted for by other factors, such as a change in medical status, lifestyle, or the natural progression of the disorder
- It is assumed that there has been a prior positive response to treatment

In addition to A, either B or C (or both) need to be satisfied:

B. Persisting (although not immediate) **paradoxical response to treatment**: RLS symptom severity increases some time after a dose increase and improves some time after a dose decrease.

C. Earlier onset of symptoms:
- An earlier onset by at least 4 hours OR
- An earlier onset (between 2 and 4 hours) occurs with one of the following compared with symptom status before treatment:
  - Shorter latency to symptoms when at rest
  - Extension of symptoms to other body parts
  - Greater intensity of symptoms or increase in periodic limb movements if measured by polysomnography or the suggested immobilization test
  - Shorter duration of relief from treatment

* Augmentation requires that criteria A + B, A + C, or A + (B + C) be met.

Garcia-Borreguero D, et al. *Sleep Med.* 2007;8:520-530.

short half-life of 1.5 hours and an effective duration of about 2 to 3 hours. The slow-release formulations of L-dopa (CR) may last 4 to 6 hours but have a much slower onset of action.

The side effects of L-dopa are similar to the other dopamine drugs (**Table 9.2**).

The dose range of L-dopa for RLS is 50 to 200 mg per day (combined with either 10, 25, or 50 mg carbidopa or 12.5, 25, or 50 mg benserazide). Keeping the dose <200 mg per day may help prevent augmentation, but even these smaller doses have been associated with this side effect. It is therefore best to limit the use of this drug for intermittent RLS symptoms for which it can be very useful and safe.

Extending L-dopa With COMT Inhibitors

Catechol-*O*–methyl transferase (COMT) is an enzyme that is involved in the breakdown of the catecholamine neurotransmitters, dopamine, epinephrine, and norepinephrine. This enzyme also breaks down L-dopa and, in the presence of a decarboxylase inhibitor (carbidopa or benserazide), COMT becomes the major metabolizing enzyme for L-dopa.

Therefore, adding an inhibitor of COMT to the combination medication of L-dopa and carbidopa or benserazide increases the bioavailability of L-dopa by about 2-fold. The half-life of L-dopa is increased, which results in more sustained plasma levels of the drug but the peak concentration is unaltered.

There are currently two COMT inhibitors available in the United States:
- Tolcapone
- Entacapone.

While tolcapone increases the bioavailability of L-dopa 2-fold and the half-life to 3.5 hours, entacapone increases the bioavailability of L-dopa by 35% and the half-life to 2.4 hours. However, due to the 10- to 100-fold increase in fulminant liver failure caused by tolcapone, it has been withdrawn from many countries, except the United States. There is also one combination medication that contains L-dopa, carbidopa, and tolcapone.

The use of COMT inhibitors has been well established for treating Parkinson's disease. However, as the use of L-dopa is now mostly limited to treating intermittent RLS symptoms, the role of adding a COMT inhibitor is an unknown. As the addition of a COMT inhibitor does not affect the time of onset or of peak concentration, these may be useful drugs to prolong the otherwise short-lived effects of L-dopa. However, until these drugs are studied, we do not really know their efficacy for treating RLS or whether they alter L-dopa's common problem of augmentation.

■ Rebound

Rebound, first described in 1993,[19] can be a problem with many of the dopaminergic medications, especially the shorter-acting drugs. Rebound occurs when the effect of the drug wears off and RLS symptoms recur due to drug levels that are inadequate to control them. This is simply an end of the drug-dose effect.

A typical example of this phenomenon is the use of L-dopa (half-life of 1.5 hours) to treat bedtime RLS. If the drug is taken at 11 PM and the person wakes up after 3 PM, the low levels of drug left in the body are insufficient to relieve the reemerging RLS symptoms.

Rebound is easily managed. As soon as symptoms recur, patients can simply take another dose of the short-acting medication to treat these symptoms. If rebound becomes a frequent problem, it is better to change to a longer-acting drug, such as one of the dopamine agonists.

It is less common to see rebound with ropinirole (half-life of 6 hours) or pramipexole (half-life of 8 to 12 hours). However, if these drugs are given early enough in the day (before 7 PM) to treat afternoon or evening RLS, they can result in middle-of-the-night rebound symptoms. Longer half-life medications, such as currently available cabergoline—only formulated in

Europe for PD or RLS—may alleviate this problem or off-label treatment with divided doses of agonists.

■ Augmentation

Augmentation is a worsening of RLS symptoms (**Table 9.4**) caused by the drug that is being used to treat the disorder. For the most part, this problem occurs mainly with drugs that work on the dopamine system, but there have been two articles reporting augmentation with tramadol.[20,21] Usually, the worsening from augmentation occurs weeks or months after starting medication for RLS.[22]

The mechanism of augmentation is not yet understood. It may seem strange that a drug that first improves the RLS symptoms later causes worsening. Several theories exist to explain this phenomenon including downregulation of the dopamine receptors (similar to tolerance) and overstimulation of the dopamine D_1 receptors compared with D_2 receptors.[23] It is also thought that iron deficiency may be a key predisposing factor for developing augmentation by causing a reduced function of the dopamine transporter.[23]

Augmentation is Associated With Dopaminergic Drugs, Especially L-dopa

Augmentation of RLS due to L-dopa was first described and studied in 1996,[2] many years after this drug was first used to treat the disorder. This study found that 82% of RLS patients treated with L-dopa developed problems with augmentation. There was an association with dose in that augmentation occurred more readily in those who took ≥200 mg L-dopa per day. Although lower daily doses are less likely to cause augmentation, they still can cause this problem. As augmentation symptoms due to L-dopa tend to be very severe, it is recommended that L-dopa–containing drugs be used only on an intermittent basis.

Augmentation rates appear to be lower with the dopamine agonists.[24] The exact prevalence of augmentation due to dopamine agonists is still not well-known. Most of the studies have been done before the newer diagnostic criteria were developed or have not been structured (usually are too short) to capture this side effect or have required investigators to volunteer augmentation as a side effect rather than seeking it out specifically. A more recent long-term follow-up study found that 32% of those on pramipexole developed augmentation.[25] Cabergoline may have a lower rate of augmentation: <3% in one study[26] and 9% in another.[27] Rates with pergolide vary between 0% and 27%.[28-30] So far, there is little information on augmentation with ropinirole (2.3% in a recent 52-week study).[31] Because of the limitations of the data collected, it is not now possible to compare different agonists with respect to rate of augmentation.

9

The lower rates of augmentation with dopamine agonists compared with L-dopa have been attributed to their longer half-life.[28] To date, cabergoline with its >65-hour half-life seems to have the lowest incidence of augmentation. However, the long duration of this drug's action may actually treat augmentation symptoms that occur earlier in the day. Evaluating augmentation may become more difficult as agents with more sustained therapeutic levels are introduced into RLS treatment.

In addition to lower augmentation rates, the dopamine agonists tend to cause less severe symptoms compared with L-dopa. Often, the RLS symptoms just occur a few hours earlier in the day but are mild. With L-dopa, the symptoms often become so intense that patients will describe them as "incredible torture." It is common for patients to increase their dose of L-dopa to several tablets per day in a vain attempt to relieve these unbearable symptoms.

Although lower doses of L-dopa result in fewer problems with augmentation,[2] this has not yet been shown to be the case for dopamine agonists. Despite this, some experts believe that lower doses of a dopamine agonist may help decrease the incidence of augmentation.[23]

It has also been found that augmentation rates are higher in people with a family history of RLS and those who do not have neuropathy associated with their RLS.[32]

Diagnosis and Evaluation

Once the issue of augmentation is understood, most cases should be obvious once the diagnostic criteria (**Table 9.4**) are noted. The key to diagnosing augmentation is associating the worsening of symptoms with the initiation of dopamine treatment. This can be particularly difficult when the problem occurs many months after the onset of therapy.

Patients will usually complain that after the initial period of weeks to months of experiencing relief from their symptoms with dopamine medication, symptoms begin to occur at least 2 hours earlier in the day. These symptoms may become more intense, may spread to other body parts (especially the arms but expansion to all other body parts including the face is possible), and the time at rest before symptoms occur may significantly decrease. In addition, the previous dose of medication may not be as effective in decreasing symptoms or last as long. Increasing the dose may help at first, then become less effective and may lead to further augmentation symptoms. Stopping the medication will typically result in a marked increase in symptoms followed by a return to pretreatment levels after a few weeks.

Symptoms (**Table 9.2**) must be present for at least 1 week and a minimum of 5 days per week before augmentation can be diagnosed.[24] The onset of symptoms can be as soon as 1 week but typically occurs within 2 months when due to L-dopa[24] or 6 to 9 months with dopamine agonists.[24,25] One long-term study on pramipexole found that no further cases of augmentation occurred after 2.5 years.[4]

Augmentation must be differentiated from situations that may appear somewhat similar (**Table 9.5**). As RLS tends to worsen slowly with time, one must be sure that the worsening of symptoms is not due to disease progression. This can be difficult at times as the disease may progress in an erratic fashion. Generally, RLS symptoms occurring >2.5 years after the onset of therapy are much more likely to be due to disease progression. At times, the only way to decide if augmentation exists is to stop the dopamine drug and see if symptoms revert to where they were prior to treatment (which does not occur with disease progression).

Initially, rebound may be confused with augmentation in that patients complain about a worsening of symptoms despite therapy. However, rebound occurs at the end of the dose as a late effect while augmentation presents as an earlier onset of symptoms.

Tolerance shares some of the features of augmentation in that the drug effect diminishes; higher doses are needed to treat symptoms and drug responsiveness usually returns after a few weeks off the drug. Due to these similarities, it has been suggested that tolerance may in fact be a subtype of augmentation[25] caused by a similar downregulation of dopamine receptors. However, for diagnostic purposes, tolerance does not

9

TABLE 9.5 — Differential Diagnosis of Augmentation

- Natural disease progression of restless legs syndrome
- Rebound
- Tolerance
- Worsening of restless legs syndrome due to other factors

---

result in an earlier onset of RLS symptoms or expansion of symptoms to other body parts.

Worsening of symptoms due to other causes must also be ruled out. Medications (antihistamines, psychiatric medication, etc), iron deficiency, sleep deprivation, alcohol use, and vigorous exercise are among the many different causes that may exacerbate RLS. Before diagnosing augmentation, doctors should search for exacerbating factors. If the worsened RLS symptoms can be linked to one of these extrinsic factors, symptoms may be improved by simply correcting the offending cause.

Treating Augmentation

The treatment of augmentation depends upon the intensity and timing of symptoms. Most cases of augmentation due to L-dopa are so severe that only one alternative exists: Stop the medication immediately.[28] However, this must be done carefully as RLS symptoms become even more intense when L-dopa is withdrawn from someone suffering from augmentation.

Some specialists recommend starting a dopamine agonist to substitute for the L-dopa.[28] The concern with this replacement therapy is that the dopamine agonist must be titrated up slowly to prevent side effects and thus may take too long to become effective enough to cover the withdrawal symptoms. The worsening of RLS may be somewhat mitigated by slowly tapering the L-dopa (especially with larger doses) while increasing the dopamine agonist. There is some controversy about replacing one dopaminergic drug with another due to the concern of recurrent augmentation, but the risk of this does not appear that significant.[4]

An alternative approach used by many specialists is to discontinue the L-dopa abruptly and then treat the withdrawal symptoms with a potent narcotic. The augmented RLS symptoms usually return to baseline within about 3 days.[28] The narcotic may be continued for a few more weeks to cover the symptoms until the dopamine agonist is titrated to the appropriate dose. Further treatment of augmentation is discussed in Chapter 10, *Approaching the Patient With RLS*, under the heading of *Refractory Patients*.

■ Unapproved Medications for Treating RLS

This next group of drugs consists of older dopamine agonists that have been used for RLS and newer ones that are under investigation. The older dopamine agonists may never be FDA approved for RLS due to side effects or because most are already off patent.

It still may be important to be familiar with these drugs as they can be useful at times. The dopamine agonists can be divided into two groups; those that are derived from ergot alkaloids (produced by a fungus that infects rye and other plants) and those that are not related to ergots. Ropinirole, pramipexole, and rotigotine are not derived from ergot alkaloids but most of the other dopamine agonists are in this category (bromocriptine, cabergoline, lisuride, pergolide).

The ergot-derived dopamine agonists all share a common property of causing fibrosis in the abdomen, lung, and heart.[33] There are many reports of retroperitoneal fibrosis,[34,35] pleuropulmonary fibrosis (interstitial and pleural),[36,37] and cardiac fibrosis (pericardial and valvular).[38-41] In fact, due to the recent finding that the incidence of ergot-induced valvular damage is as high as 22% in one study (cabergoline and pergolide)[42] and 29% with cabergoline and 23% with pergolide in another study,[43] pergolide has been voluntarily removed from the US market. This does not appear to be a problem with the non–ergot-derived dopamine agonists as these same studies found an incidence of either 3% (with no controls)[42] or 0% (6% in controls).[43]

Until further study is done on the problem, ergot-related dopamine agonists (bromocriptine, cabergoline, and pergolide) should be used with caution with echocardiogram monitoring at regular intervals (3 to 6 months). It is thought that these ergot drugs induce fibrotic changes by activating the $5HT_{2B}$ receptors (a subtype of serotonin receptor) that stimulate fibrocytes. Therefore, ergot drugs such as lisuride and terguride that antagonize the $5HT_{2B}$ receptors may not stimulate fibrosis.[44,45] In fact, no reports of fibrotic heart damage have yet appeared for lisuride[46] despite >20 years of clinical use in the same clinical population as other ergot dopamine agonists.

For convenient reference, these drugs are listed alphabetically by generic name, although they differ in the amount of evidence that supports their use in RLS.

Apomorphine

This non–ergot-related drug is a derivative of morphine that has both dopamine agonist and opioid properties and is only approved for use in Parkinson's disease.[47] A few studies have demonstrated its efficacy in selected cases.[48,49]

Apomorphine is quite different from all of the other dopamine agonists in that it is administered by subcutaneous injection. As such, it is extremely fast acting This drug should not be given without an antiemetic, as nausea and vomiting are common and significant problems.

Bromocriptine

This ergot-derived drug, approved for use in prolactin-producing pituitary tumors and Parkinson's disease, was the first dopamine agonist employed to treat RLS. First described for treating RLS by Sevket Akpinar in 1982,[1] there are only a few studies describing its efficacy for treating RLS.[50-52]

Cabergoline

This is one of the newer ergot-derived dopamine agonist drugs. It is unique in that it has a very long half-life of >65 hours. Studies performed in Europe have demonstrated cabergoline's efficacy and safety for RLS. [53,54]

A benefit of this drug includes its once-daily dosing, which is ideal for patients with severe RLS who otherwise need up to three doses of currently available drugs. In addition, possibly due to its long duration, augmentation rates appear to be quite low. Its side effect profile is similar to that of other dopamine agonists, although one recent study that compared it with L-dopa found that it has a higher incidence of adverse reactions.[55] Like other ergot-derived drugs, it has been implicated in causing fibrosis.

Cabergoline is metabolized in the liver and has the very long half-life of >65 hours. Its onset of action is about 1 to 3 hours. It is given once daily in the evening starting at 0.25 to 0.5 mg and increased on a weekly basis by 0.25 to 0.5 mg, to a maximum dose of 4 mg. The average effective dose is about 2 mg.

Lisuride

This drug, which is not available in the United States, is approved in Europe to treat Parkinson's disease, hyperprolactinemia, and migraine headaches (off label). Lisuride is an ergot-related dopamine agonist. Due to its short half-life and variable bioavailability, this drug is better suited to treat RLS by the transdermal route. Despite its being an ergot-related dopamine drug, it does not appear to cause fibrotic changes, as do the others in this class (see discussion above). There are two studies in RLS conducted by the same investigator.[56,57]

Pergolide

This ergot-derived dopamine agonist has recently been voluntarily withdrawn from the US drug market due to its association with fibrotic heart valve damage (see above); as of this writing, it is still available in

Europe. Many studies have found it to be an effective treatment for RLS when tolerated.[58-61]

Piribedil

Piribedil is a non–ergot-derived dopamine agonist that is not available in the United States but approved elsewhere for Parkinson's disease, cognitive disorders, and treatment of retinal ischemic manifestations. It is generally prescribed in its slow-release form. There is only one study that examined the use of piribedil in RLS.[62]

Rotigotine

Rotigotine is currently under evaluation in the United States and Europe for RLS but is approved in the United States and Europe for Parkinson's disease. Due to its very low oral bioavailability from an extensive first-pass effect, this non–ergot-derived dopamine agonist is given by the transdermal route. After the patch is applied, there is a lag time of about 2 to 3 hours before the drug reaches the systemic circulation and about 24 hours until it reaches peak concentrations. Plasma levels are stable at 2 to 3 days. Rotigotine is metabolized in the liver, then excreted mostly through the kidneys.

To date, only two studies have been published assessing the use of this drug for RLS. The first pilot study randomized subjects with moderate to severe RLS to three patch doses: 0.5 mg, 1 mg, and 2 mg daily for 1 week.[63] All doses improved RLS symptoms, with the 2-mg dose being the most effective. The second study examined the dose-response curve with respect to safety and tolerability and optimum dosing of the rotigotine patch.[64] Using five patch doses (0.5, 1, 2, 3, and 4 mg), this study found that the optimal dose range was 1 to 3 mg, as the lowest dose of 0.5 mg was not effective and there was no additional benefit with the highest dose of 4 mg.

Side effects were mild, with nausea, vomiting, and skin irritation at the application site being the more common problems. Several additional large-scale clinical trials have been completed and reported in abstract that should further define its long-term efficacy and safety for RLS.

Terguride

Terguride is a partial dopamine agonist (ergot-derived) that is not available in the United States and is approved to treat hyperprolactinemia. It has a half-life of 4.3 hours and comes to peak concentration in 1 hour.[65] Side effects are similar to those of other dopamine agonists.

Only one study has assessed terguride for treating RLS.[66]

Anticonvulsants   9

Although not approved for RLS, anticonvulsant drugs (**Table 9**.6) were the third class of drugs used for RLS in modern times (after sedative hypnotics and dopaminergics), with the first report describing carbamazepine in 1983,[67] shortly after the account of L-dopa's use for RLS. Typically, anticonvulsants are moderately effective for RLS symptoms and are considered second-line drugs.[3] Sedation, which often carries over to the next day, tends to be their major limitation. However, when the sedation occurs only at bedtime, it may actually be an advantage in using these drugs.

In addition, anticonvulsants have been suggested to be particularly useful for painful RLS symptoms or for neuropathies that are often associated with RLS. Although most of these drugs may be efficacious for relieving RLS symptoms, the majority of studies have examined gabapentin. In these patients, some of these drugs can be used for approved indications of pain relief or for RLS associated with peripheral neuropathies.

TABLE 9.6 — Anticonvulsant Drugs	
Anticonvulsant	**Individual Dose Range (mg)**
Carbamazepine	100-400, up to 3×/day
Gabapentin	100-900, up to 3×/day
Lamotrigine	25-250, up to 2×/day
Levetiracetam	250-1500, up to 2×/day
Oxcarbazepine	150-1200, up to 2×/day
Pregabalin	25-200, up to 3×/day or 75-300, up to 2×/day
Tiagabine	2-16, up to 2×/day
Topiramate	25-200, up to 2×/day
Valproic acid	250-500, up to 2-3×/day
Zonisamide	100-600, once daily

■ Gabapentin

Gabapentin was first studied in RLS in 1996 in an open trial of 16 subjects and found to be an effective therapy.[68] Further case studies confirmed its efficacy for both RLS and PLMS in doses between 300 and 1200 mg/day but did not find that it helped sleep parameters (possibly due to only mildly impaired sleep prior to treatment).[69] A subsequent larger and double-blinded study found the drug to be effective for RLS and PLMS and furthermore that sleep parameters (increased total sleep time, sleep efficiency, slow-wave sleep, and decreased stage 1 sleep) were improved at a mean effective dose of 1855 mg/day.[70] That study also found that subjects with increased symptoms of pain benefited the most from gabapentin. This is in keeping with this drug's effect on neuropathic pain.

The most recent study compared gabapentin with ropinirole in an open trial and determined that both drugs are equally effective and well tolerated.[71] However, doses were smaller (300-1200 mg/day) than in other studies and those typically used in practice where sedation often proves troublesome. Other studies (discussed in Chapter 11, *Special Considerations*) have demonstrated its benefit for dialysis patients with RLS.[72,73]

Gabapentin, a structural analogue of γ-aminobutyric acid (GABA) that is an inhibitory neurotransmitter in the CNS, is approved in the United States for the treatment of epilepsy and postherpetic neuralgia; however, its mechanism of action is unknown. Side effects include sedation and drowsiness (the most common reasons to discontinue use), dizziness, and peripheral edema. The half-life is about 5 to 7 hours, and it is eliminated unaltered by the kidneys.

Typically, gabapentin is started at 300 mg (although 100 mg can be initiated in elderly or sensitive patients), 2 to 3 hours before symptoms usually occur up to three times daily. The dose may be titrated by 100- to 300-mg increments every 3 to 7 days until symptoms are relieved. Although some people are responsive to lower doses of 300 mg, most require 1200 mg to 2000 mg daily. Since gabapentin is eliminated unaltered through the kidneys, patients with renal impairment need lower doses and it should be titrated more gradually.

■ Other Anticonvulsants

Most of the other anticonvulsants have been used in varying degrees for RLS (**Table 9.6**). They can all be considered second-line agents and all RLS use is off-label. Although there is much less experience with these other drugs, any of them may prove more efficacious or tolerable in given individuals. Therefore, it is often worth trying several in this class until one is found that suits the patient. Some of the newer ones (such as pregabalin) may have less sedation as an unwanted reaction. These medications are also listed alphabetically.

Carbamazepine

As noted,[67] this was the second drug and first anticonvulsant studied for RLS. It has not received too much more attention (except for three studies by the same group[74-76]) as many newer anticonvulsants have since been developed. It is approved in the United States for use in epilepsy and trigeminal neuralgia.

Common side effects include dizziness, drowsiness, unsteadiness, nausea, and vomiting. Rare but severe dermatologic reactions, including toxic epidermal necrolysis and Stevens-Johnson syndrome, may occur as may rare cases of pancytopenia or hepatic failure that require frequent monitoring of blood tests.

The drug is metabolized in the liver and has an initial half-life of 25 to 65 hours, decreasing to 12 to 17 hours with repeated doses. Due to its metabolism by the cytochrome P450 system, it may interact with many other drugs. One study[67] found that doses of 800 to 1000 mg were more effective than lower doses. However, the other studies found improvement compared with placebo using more limited doses of 100 to 300 mg.

Lamotrigine

This drug, approved in the United States for epilepsy and bipolar disorder, is an antiepileptic drug of the phenyltriazine class, chemically unrelated to existing antiepileptic drugs. There is one pilot study that demonstrated some benefit of lamotrigine in three out of four subjects with RLS (one withdrew due to dizziness).[77]

Levetiracetam

Levetiracetam is approved in the United States for epilepsy. There is only one article examining this drug in two patients with RLS.[78] Both patients had RLS symptoms refractory to dopamine agonists, but responded to 500-1000 mg of levetiracetam at bedtime and sustained this benefit for >21 months.

Oxcarbazepine

This drug is approved in the United States for epilepsy. There is only one article discussing the dosing of oxcarbazepine for RLS; 150 mg twice daily was used to successfully treat a case of paroxetine-induced RLS.[79]

Pregabalin

Pregabalin was designed to be a more potent successor to gabapentin. It is approved in the United States for epilepsy, postherpetic neuralgia, and neuropathic pain associated with diabetic peripheral neuropathy. Only one open-label study has been published on pregabalin; it was found to be effective for 16 of 19 patients with RLS (16 of whom also had a painful neuropathy).[80] The average dose was 305 mg.

Topiramate

Topiramate is approved in the United States for use in epilepsy and for prophylaxis of migraine headaches. There has been only one study published on the use of topiramate in RLS[81] that found it to be an effective treatment. The mean effective dose was established at 42 mg with a range of 25 to 100 mg.

Valproic Acid

This drug is approved in the United States for use in epilepsy. At present, only one study has examined the use of this drug for RLS.[82] This study compared valproic acid (600 mg) and L-dopa/benserazide (200/50), using a placebo-controlled, crossover, double-blind method and found no major difference between the efficacy of these drugs over a 3-week test period. However, they found that the decrease in intensity and duration of RLS symptoms was more pronounced with valproic acid than with L-dopa.

Opioids

Opioids were the first documented drugs prescribed for RLS for a woman with RLS whom Sir Thomas Willis effectively treated in 1672. Since Willis's description and then other successful treatment of RLS in 1685, several centuries passed before the use of opioids for RLS was rediscovered. The next known documentation of the benefit of opioids (except for Karl Ekbom in 1960[83] and Sevket Akpinar in 1982,[1] who anecdotally noted that RLS responds to opioids) occurred in 1984 (2 years after L-dopa and 1 year after carbamazepine) with the report of three patients who responded well to treatment with low doses of opioids (methadone 10 mg or oxycodone 2.5 mg at bedtime).[84]

The often dramatic response of RLS to opioids led several investigators to speculate that RLS may be in part due to impairment in the function of the endogenous opiate system.[85,86] The role of the endogenous opiate system was further investigated with studies demonstrating that these drugs helped RLS symptoms and that naloxone could reverse this therapeutic action but had no effect on its own or after a dopamine agonist.[87-89] Interestingly, the effect of opioids on RLS may be in part due to their action on the dopaminergic system as dopamine receptor antagonists block their therapeutic actions on RLS.[90]

■ Wide Variety of Formulations

There are many different opioids available and for purposes of treating RLS, they are often divided according to their potency into three categories: low, medium, and high (**Table 9**.7). Dosing guidelines vary with the specific drugs (**Table 9**.7). There are very few published data on the use of this class of medication for patients with RLS and none is approved to treat RLS. Some may be prescribed for the approved indications of pain when this occurs as a component of the RLS treatment.

Due to their potential for tolerance and dependence, these drugs are not considered to be a first-line treatment for RLS. However, they can be valuable medications for those who cannot tolerate or do not improve on the dopamine agonists or anticonvulsants. For many severe RLS sufferers, opioids may provide their only source of relief. As these medications tend to onset quickly (usually within 10 to 15 minutes), they are very useful for treating unexpected episodes of RLS on an intermittent basis where there is no risk of tolerance or dependence.

Choosing the correct opioid from the many available may seem difficult, but with understanding of the drugs, this decision may be easier. Typically, the lowest dose and least potent of these drugs should be tried first, then increased as necessary.

Many of these opioid analgesics are combined with acetaminophen, aspirin, or ibuprofen. Although these additives help reduce pain, they have no therapeutic effect on RLS. Therefore, they can only cause adverse effects without adding any positive benefits and should be avoided when possible. *If possible, opioid analgesics should be chosen in their pure form without any unhelpful (for RLS) additives.*

Side Effects of Opioids

Adverse reactions to opioids tend to be similar and include light-headedness, dizziness, sedation, constipation, nausea, and vomiting. These side effects tend to be dose dependent and are more common among the more potent opioids. Another concern with the more potent opioids is respiratory depression (especially in patients with COPD) and worsening of the very common disorder, obstructive sleep apnea.

TABLE 9.7 — Opioid Drugs

Drug Name	Usual Dose Range for RLS	Potency for Treating RLS
Codeine	15-60 mg q 4-6 hours	Low
Fentanyl	12.5-25 mcg/hour patch	High
Hydrocodone	2.5-10 mg q 4-6 hours	Medium
Hydromorphone	2-8 mg q 4-6 hours	High
Levorphanol	2-4 mg q 6-8 hours	High
Meperidine, oral	50-300 mg q 3-4 hours	Low
Methadone	5-10 mg q 8 hours	High
Morphine	5-10 mg q 4-6 hours	High
Morphine (controlled-release)	15-30 mg q 12 hours	High
Oxycodone	2.5-10 mg q 4-8 hours	High
Oxycodone (sustained-release)	10-40 q 12 hours	High

Oxymorphone	2.5-5 mg q 4-6 hours	High
Oxymorphone (extended-release)	5-10 mg q 12 hours	High
Pentazocine	50-100 mg q 3-4 hours	Low
Propoxyphene	65-100 mg q 3-4 hours	Low
Tramadol	50-100 mg q 6 hours	Medium
Tramadol (extended-release)	100-300 mg daily	Medium

9

Every drug in this class may produce tolerance and dependence when used for chronic therapy. In addition, addiction can occur readily with these drugs in susceptible people. Patients should be monitored closely for escalating use of these drugs and carefully managed when this occurs.

- ### Low-Potency Opioids

This class includes codeine, meperidine (oral), pentazocine, and propoxyphene. Due to their low potency, these drugs have more leeway than the more potent opioids for causing tolerance and dependence, and they have fewer and less severe side effects. They are very suitable for treating milder RLS symptoms and should be tried before employing the more potent agents.

Codeine

Few studies have evaluated codeine for treating RLS. One study looked retrospectively at people with RLS who used various opioids including codeine (65 to 100 mg) for long-term use.[91] Just as in clinical practice, these investigators found codeine to be effective in 24 patients for long-term use. Another study prospectively administered codeine (30 to 120 mg/day in divided doses) to two subjects who found that the drug improved their RLS symptoms.[87]

Propoxyphene

There are no trials of this drug for RLS patients but the retrospective review noted earlier[91] for codeine also found long-term effectiveness of propoxyphene (65 to 100 mg) for RLS in 25 patients. There is also one case report of a patient who controlled his symptoms with propoxyphene for 5 years[85] and another article that showed benefit prospectively giving the drug (130 to 260 mg/day in divided doses) to three subjects.[87]

■ Medium-Potency Opioids

This class includes the popular drug hydrocodone and the somewhat hard to classify drug tramadol. These drugs are reasonably similar in potency both for pain and for RLS management.

Hydrocodone

This opioid has never been studied for treating RLS and no case reports exist for this use. However, as it is a popular drug that most physicians in the United States are quite comfortable using, it is often used to treat RLS symptoms. The problem with using this drug chronically for RLS is that it is always manufactured in combination with a non-narcotic opioid analgesic (acetaminophen, aspirin, or ibuprofen). As such, these additives only increase the risk of side effects without the possibility of benefits for treating RLS. Hydrocodone can be effective in the range of 2.5 mg to 10 mg.

Tramadol

Similar to the opioids, this synthetic opioidlike drug is approved only for the short-term management of acute pain. Although often classified as an opioid, it is considered to be an atypical central-acting opioid-like drug. It is not clear exactly how this drug controls pain as it binds very weakly to the μ-opioid receptors (that are responsible for opioid's antinociceptive effects) and its effects are only partially blocked by naloxone. Its analgesic effects may be due in part from its weak inhibition of the reuptake of norepinephrine and serotonin.[92]

This different action of tramadol may account for its lower potential for abuse.[93-95] For this reason, this drug may be a reasonable choice for treating either pain or RLS. Common side effects include nausea, vomiting, sweating, and dizziness, but these occur much less frequently and less severely than with opioids. This drug is also known to lower the seizure threshold. As noted earlier, recent reports have found that tramadol is the only nondopaminergic drug to cause augmentation.[20,21]

Only one study has examined the use of tramadol for RLS in a long-term (15-24 months) open trial.[96] They found this drug to be very effective at 50-150 mg in 10 of 12 subjects.

■ High-Potency Opioids

This class includes the transdermal patch fentanyl, hydromorphone, levorphanol, methadone, morphine, oxycodone, and oxymorphone. *Since this group contains the most potent opioids that have the highest risk of tolerance, dependence, and respiratory depression, they should be prescribed with caution and only by physicians who are very familiar with their use.*

These medications are typically considered the drugs of last choice and are used when all of the other drugs have failed to relieve the RLS symptoms. However, since they are often the only drugs left that can provide relief and are reasonably safe when appropriately monitored, they should not be withheld due to their stigma as dangerous and addicting narcotics. In the absence of a history of substance abuse, it is very unusual for an RLS patient to become tolerant or dependent (except for RLS relief) on these drugs.

Fentanyl Transdermal Patches

This potent opioid, which is approved in the United States only for use in chronic pain, has the unique delivery system of a transdermal patch. There are currently no studies or reports on this drug for its use in RLS. Some specialists prescribe this drug for an occasional case of severe RLS that occurs around the clock and needs continuous treatment.

Fentanyl should be started at its lowest dose of 12.5 mcg/hour (one patch every 3 days), and increased after 6 days to 25 mcg/hour, if necessary.

Hydromorphone, Levorphanol, and Oxymorphone

There are no studies or case reports on these three very potent opioids that are approved in the United States only for relief of moderate to severe pain. There is little experience with these medications for RLS; however, some physicians who are familiar with them have found that they are quite effective at relieving RLS symptoms. Since oxymorphone has just been released in the United States in its oral form, experience with this drug for any purpose is minimal.

Methadone

This drug is approved for treating severe pain and for narcotic addiction detoxification and maintenance. Several reports found this drug to be beneficial for treating RLS. One study describes a patient who benefited from 10 mg at bedtime and worsened when the dose was reduced.[84] Another study prospectively gave methadone (5-20 mg/day, usually in 2 divided doses) to two subjects and found it to be effective.[87] Eight further patients benefiting from the long-term use of methadone 10 mg were noted in a retrospective review.[91] The most recent study retrospectively reviewed 29 patients in whom dopaminergic therapy failed; they then took methadone (average dose was 16 mg/day and range was 5-40 mg/day, usually in 2 equal doses) and found that 17 of them remained on the drug with marked reduction in their RLS symptoms for an average of 23 months.[97] Adverse events were mild to moderate and similar to those seen with opioids in general; no subjects developed tolerance.

Despite the lack of proper medical studies to determine the efficacy, safety, and dosing of this drug, there is a significant cadre of RLS specialists who preferentially use methadone to treat refractory or severe RLS cases. This is due to several properties of methadone that make it quite useful for managing RLS.

Due to its long half-life, methadone can relieve pain for 8 to 12 hours.[98] Similarly, it tends to eliminate RLS symptoms longer than most drugs, allowing for two to three doses per day to be effective. Its use for narcotic addiction supports its decreased abuse potential compared with other opioids.[99] Methadone may cause less tolerance than other opioids as it does not cause intracellular forskolin-stimulated cAMP accumulation, a mechanism thought to contribute to opioid tolerance.[100]

Morphine

This drug is approved in the United States only for the treatment of moderate to severe pain. It is not commonly employed for treating RLS; however, there are two articles that report using it for RLS.[101,102]

Oxycodone

This drug is approved in the United States only for the treatment of moderate to severe pain. A few studies have been done to evaluate the treatment of RLS with oxycodone. The first study reports two cases that responded very well to oxycodone at 2.5 mg.[84] The next study retrospectively reviewed 30 patients who did well with oxycodone 5 mg for long-term therapy.[91] The last study, which is a double-blind, placebo, cross-over protocol, demonstrated that flexible dosing of oxycodone 5-25 mg/day (taken in two to three divided doses) significantly improved all RLS symptoms.[103] The average dose was between 10 and 15 mg/day.

Sedative Hypnotics

Although these drugs were among the first used and reported on (in 1979) for treating RLS,[104] there is considerable controversy about whether they actually relieve RLS symptoms. Most RLS experts use these drugs sparingly to treat RLS symptoms, for which they are not approved, but rather to treat the insomnia associated with RLS (for which most are approved).

The early studies that were mostly open-label protocols reported dramatic improvements with these drugs (eg, clonazepam). Sleep disruption is the major complaint of RLS sufferers[105] and the sedative-hypnotic drugs address this problem extremely well. It is not entirely clear from these early reports whether the RLS symptoms were more bedtime related or were also prominent earlier in the day and whether the daytime symptoms were equally relieved.

The second concern when assessing the open-label studies is the strong placebo effect in RLS studies. This placebo effect may account for much of the relief of any daytime symptoms attributed to the benzodiazepines. Even in the placebo-controlled trials, the marked improvement of disruptive sleep patterns due to the use of these drugs and resultant increased daytime well-being may decrease the perception of bothersome daytime RLS symptoms.

Another concern about the use of sedative hypnotics (especially with their daytime use or with the bedtime use of long-acting ones that may spill over into the next day) is that they have a potential for worsening daytime RLS symptoms and increasing the risk of accidents from activities that require vigilance. It is well accepted that RLS symptoms increase with both physical and mental rest[105] so that drugs that cause sedation may actually increase RLS symptoms. One study found that intravenous administration of diphenhydramine 25 mg or lorazepam 0.5 mg to 12 RLS patients who were adequately treated with dopamine agonists caused both similar and severe exacerbation of their otherwise controlled RLS symptoms.[106]

However, the real goal of physicians is to make patients feel better. If these drugs do accomplish this goal for RLS sufferers, they should be considered, especially when other drugs have not been helpful. Furthermore, a significant group of RLS sufferers do state that the sedative-hypnotic drugs relieve their symptoms. Additionally, these drugs markedly decrease awakenings and stage 1 sleep from PLM,[107] which are so common in RLS sufferers, which may be another benefit from their use (see *Chapter 11*).

It is not uncommon for long-time RLS sufferers to have continued insomnia even after their symptoms have been resolved by treatment. After years of not sleeping well, they typically develop a conditioned insomnia. The use of sedative-hypnotic drugs may be invaluable to break this poor sleep cycle.

However, when choosing a sedative hypnotic, it is generally best to select one that has a quick onset to promote sleep initiation and a relatively short half-life to prevent daytime sleepiness or drowsiness that in turn may promote increased RLS symptoms (**Table 9.8**). For chronic daily use, the nonbenzodiazepines (**Table 9.9**) are far more preferred due to their decreased side effect profile and markedly decreased risk of tolerance and dependence.

■ Benzodiazepines

This group comprises several drugs that share similarities and are marketed either as hypnotics for inducing sleep or to treat anxiety (**Table 9.8**). Despite being approved and marketed only as sedatives, some of these drugs may be suitable for use as hypnotics. The following discussion will review the literature on the use of these medications for treating RLS. Drugs are listed alphabetically.

Alprazolam

An open-label study examined alprazolam at 0.5 mg to 1 mg at bedtime in 10 subjects with RLS.[108] They found that eight of their 10 patients improved on the alprazolam. One patient stated that taking 0.5 mg of

TABLE 9.8 — Benzodiazepines (Hypnotics and Sedatives)

Generic Drug Name	Half-Life (hours)	Individual Dose Range (mg)	Approved as a Hypnotic for Sleep
Alprazolam	6-12	0.25-1	No
Clonazepam	30-40	0.5-2	No
Clorazepate	48	7.5-30	No
Chlordiazepoxide	7-48	2-25	No
Diazepam	24-100	2-10	No
Estazolam	10-24	0.5-2	Yes
Flurazepam	47-100	15-30	Yes
Lorazepam	10-20	0.5-2	No
Oxazapam	8	10-30	No
Quazepam	39-73	7.5-30	Yes
Temazepam	9.5-12.5	7.5-30	Yes
Triazolam	1.5-5.5	0.125-0.5	Yes

9

TABLE 9.9 — Nonbenzodiazepine Hypnotics		
Generic Drug Name	Half-Life (hours)	Individual Dose Range (mg)
Ramelteon	1-2.6	8
Eszopiclone	6	1-3
Zaleplon	1	10-20
Zolpidem	2.5	2.5-10
Zolpidem (slow-release)	2.8	6.25-12.5

the drug before going to the theater provided her with relief throughout the entire evening.

Clonazepam

The first report on the use of this drug for RLS was a letter to the editor in 1979 that described two people who benefited greatly from the bedtime and evening use of clonazepam 0.5-1 mg.[104] This was followed by another letter to the editor that reported on three more people who benefited from taking clonazepam 0.5 mg one to three times daily.[109] The first double-blind crossover trial of clonazepam in RLS found it to be more effective on six subjects compared with placebo and quite safe to use.[110] They also examined the use of vibration to the leg and did not find it significantly effective.

However, the next study, also a placebo-controlled, double-blind, crossover study, did not find clonazepam to be more effective than placebo on six subjects.[111] This article clearly adds to the controversy about whether clonazepam relieves RLS symptoms or merely helps RLS patients sleep better.

Clonazepam is a readily available and inexpensive drug and as such has a particular physician following for treating RLS. As noted above, it clearly resolves the insomnia associated with RLS and improves well-being in people who are suffering prior to treatment.

The concern with this drug is that it has a 30 to 40 hour half-life, which may easily result in next-day sedation, especially when taken for several nights consecutively. This daytime sedation is often not apparent to the patient especially when compared with their previous RLS-induced sleep-deprived state. As other shorter-acting sedative hypnotics have been shown to be effective for RLS (see below), there are alternatives that may be safer and inexpensive.

In addition, clonazepam, like other benzodiazepines, may cause tolerance and dependence when used on a daily basis. Using nonbenzodiazepines dramatically diminishes this risk.

Temazepam

No studies have yet evaluated this drug for RLS. However, one study showed the efficacy of temazepam for PLM.[107]

Triazolam

There is one report of triazolam 0.25 mg taken at bedtime helping one patient with RLS for 6 months.[112] This patient stopped the drug and experienced recurrence of her symptoms within 48 hours.

There are two articles demonstrating the benefits of triazolam[113,114] for PLM. These studies have show improvements in sleep architecture by increasing total sleep time, decreasing the number of awakenings and arousals, decreasing stage 1 sleep while increasing stage 2 sleep, and increasing sleep efficiency. Additionally, daytime sleepiness was diminished. Triazolam did not decrease the PLM, but it did markedly decrease the arousals and awakenings from the PLM.

Triazolam has a quick onset of action and a short half-life of 1.5 to 5.5 hours that limits next-day drowsiness. Unfortunately, this drug has been associated with a significant degree of retrograde amnesia and rebound insomnia.

■ **Nonbenzodiazepines**

Most sleep specialists prefer using this class of drugs for treating insomnia. They have a short half-life and are associated with a limited degree of dependence or tolerance. There is only one study for RLS with zolpidem, which is discussed below. However, any of these drugs may be beneficial to help RLS patients fall asleep, whether the insomnia is due to RLS symptoms.

Eszopiclone and Zaleplon

These two drugs fill some of the gaps that are not fully covered by zolpidem therapy. Although there are no studies of these drugs for RLS, it is likely that they may work fairly similarly to zolpidem.

Ramelteon

This drug is very different from all of the other hypnotic drugs discussed. It does not act upon the GABA receptors that help promote sleep but rather on the melatonin receptors. This drug, which has relatively few side effects, is indicated for sleep-onset insomnia, since its effects on improving sleep maintenance are much less pronounced.[115]

Zolpidem

This drug was studied for RLS in one open-label prospective trial on eight subjects who were unresponsive to or could not tolerate L-dopa and benzodiazepines.[116] They found that all patients had complete relief from their RLS symptoms within an average of 4 days of starting zolpidem 10 mg that lasted 12 to 30 months with no relapses or side effects.

Zolpidem has a quick onset of action and a short half-life of 2.5 hours. It has been associated with abnormal sleep-related behaviors, such as sleep-walking, sleep-talking, or a sleep-related eating disorder,[117] but otherwise has been well tolerated. There is a controlled-release version of this drug that increases the half-life to 2.8 hours.

Other Pharmacologic Options

These other drugs do not fit into the four major categories of drugs that are commonly used to treat RLS. In addition, there is very little literature or experience to support the use of these drugs. However, in cases where the standard drugs are not effective or tolerated, these drugs may be considered. They include: amantadine,[118] botulinum toxin type-A,[119] clonidine,[120-125] and propranolol.[126-130]

Vitamins and minerals have also been suggested for RLS therapy. These include: Vitamin B_{12}[131,132] vitamin E,[133,134] folic acid,[131,132,135,136] and magnesium.[137-139] However, further evidence is necessary before these supplements can be recommended for treating RLS.

Surgery

No studies have been performed using this modality. However, several reports describe worsening of RLS after surgery. These include worsening of RLS after gastric surgery,[140] after above-knee leg amputation,[141] after heart surgery,[142] and after lung surgery.[143] The cause of surgery exacerbating RLS is unknown and may be due to multiple factors. However, it is interesting to note that there are many anecdotal reports of worsening or triggering of RLS after trauma or injury (especially spine or back related).[144] These have not been validated by formal epidemiologic studies.

There is clear evidence for improvement of the secondary RLS associated with end-stage renal disease with kidney transplantation.[145,146] RLS symptoms disappeared within 1 to 21 days of the transplant, with four of 11 patients remaining symptom-free up to 9 years, three patients had gradual reemergence of mild symptoms, and three patients in whom their transplants failed developed recurrence of RLS symptoms at their previous severity within 10 days to 2 months.

Various other surgeries have limited evidence for ameliorating RLS. These include one case report of RLS symptoms being immediately relieved postoperatively in the contralateral limbs after undergoing pallidotomy for Parkinson's disease.[147] Another study reported on six advanced Parkinson's disease patients who underwent bilateral subthalamic nucleus deep brain stimulation surgery and showed marked improvement in their RLS symptoms postoperatively.[148] However, in a study that implanted deep brain stimulators into the ventralis intermedius nucleus of the thalamus in nine subjects for essential tremor noted that although the tremor was improved, there was no change in the concomitant RLS symptoms.[149]

REFERENCES

1. Akpinar S. Treatment of restless legs syndrome with levodopa plus benserazide. *Arch Neurol*. 1982;39:739.
2. Allen RP, Earley CJ. Augmentation of the restless legs syndrome with carbidopa/levodopa. *Sleep*. 1996;19:205-213.
3. Silber MH, Ehrenberg BL, Allen RP, et al; Medical Advisory Board of the Restless Legs Syndrome Foundation. An algorithm for the management of restless legs syndrome. *Mayo Clin Proc*. 2004;79:916-922.
4. Silber MH, Girish M, Izurieta R. Pramipexole in the management of restless legs syndrome: an extended study. *Sleep*. 2003;26:819-821.
5. Partinen M, Hirvonen K, Jama L, et al. Efficacy and safety of pramipexole in idiopathic restless legs syndrome: a polysomnographic dose-finding study—the PRELUDE study. *Sleep Med*. 2006;7:407-417.
6. Trenkwalder C, Stiasny-Kolster K, Kupsch A, Oertel WH, Koester J, Reess J. Controlled withdrawal of pramipexole after 6 months of open-label treatment in patients with restless legs syndrome. *Mov Disord*. 2006;21:1404-1410.
7. Winkelman JW, Sethi KD, Kushida CA, et al. Efficacy and safety of pramipexole in restless legs syndrome. *Neurology*. 2006;67:1034-1039.

8. Montplaisir J, Fantini ML, Desautels A, Michaud M, Petit D, Filipini D. Long-term treatment with pramipexole in restless legs syndrome. *Eur J Neurol*. 2006;13:1306-1311.

9. Oertel WH, Stiasny-Kolster K, Bergtholdt B, et al. Pramipexole RLS Study Group. Efficacy of pramipexole in restless legs syndrome: a six-week, multicenter, randomized, double-blind study (effect-RLS study). *Mov Disord*. 2007;22:213-219.

10. Trenkwalder C, Garcia-Borreguero D, Montagna P, et al. Therapy with Ropiunirole; Efficacy and Tolerability in RLS 1 Study Group. Ropinirole in the treatment of restless legs syndrome: results from the TREAT RLS 1 study, a 12 week, randomised, placebo controlled study in 10 European countries. *J Neurol Neurosurg Psychiatry*. 2004;75:92-97.

11. Walters AS, Ondo WG, Dreykluft T, Grunstein R, Lee D, Sethi K; TREAT RLS 2 (Therapy with Ropinirole: Efficacy And Tolerability in RLS 2) Study Group. Ropinirole is effective in the treatment of restless legs syndrome. TREAT RLS 2: a 12-week, double-blind, randomized, parallel-group, placebo-controlled study. *Mov Disord*. 2004;19:1414-1423.

12. Allen R, Becker PM, Bogan R, et al. Ropinirole decreases periodic leg movements and improves sleep parameters in patients with restless legs syndrome. *Sleep*. 2004;27:907-914.

13. Bogan RK, Fry JM, Schmidt MH, Carson SW, Ritchie SY; TREAT RLS US Study Group. Ropinirole in the treatment of patients with restless legs syndrome: a US-based randomized, double-blind, placebo-controlled clinical trial. *Mayo Clin Proc*. 2006;81:17-27.

14. Tippmann-Peikert M, Park JG, Boeve BF, Shepard JW, Silber MH. Pathologic gambling in patients with restless legs syndrome treated with dopaminergic agonists. *Neurology*. 2007;68:301-303.

15. Quickfall J, Suchowersky O. Pathological gambling associated with dopamine agonist use in restless legs syndrome. *Parkinsonism Relat Disord*. 2007 Jan 29; Epub ahead of print.

16. Dodd ML, Klos KJ, Bower JH, Geda YE, Josephs KA, Ahlskog JE. Pathological gambling caused by drugs used to treat Parkinson disease. *Arch Neurol*. 2005;62:1377-1381.

17. Nirenberg MJ, Waters C. Compulsive eating and weight gain related to dopamine agonist use. *Mov Disord*. 2006;21:524-329.

18. Weintraub D, Siderowt AD, Potenza MN, et al. Association of dopamine agonist use with impulse control disorders in Parkinson disease. *Arch Neurol*. 2006;63:969-973.

19. Guilleminault C, Cetel M, Philip P. Dopaminergic treatment of restless legs and rebound phenomenon. *Neurology*. 1993;43:445.

20. Earley CJ, Allen RP. Restless legs syndrome augmentation associated with tramadol. *Sleep Med*. 2006;7:592-593.

21. Vetrugno R, La Morgia C, D'Angelo R, et al. Augmentation of restless legs syndrome with long-term tramadol treatment. *Mov Disord*. 2007;22:424-427.

22. Garcia-Borreguero D, Allen RP, Kohnen R, et al. On behalf of the International Restless Legs Syndrome Study Group (IRLSSG). Diagnostic standards for dopaminergic augmentation of restless legs syndrome: report from a world association of sleep medicine - international restless legs syndrome study group consensus conference at the max planck institute. *Sleep Med*. 2007;8:520-530.

23. Paulus W, Trenkwalder C. Less is more: pathophysiology of dopaminergic-therapy-related augmentation in restless legs syndrome. *Lancet Neurol*. 2006;5:878-886.

24. Allen RP, Picchietti D, Hening WA, Trenkwalder C, Walters AS, Montplaisi J; Restless Legs Syndrome Diagnosis and Epidemiology workshop at the National Institutes of Health; International Restless Legs Syndrome Study Group. Restless legs syndrome: diagnostic criteria, special considerations, and epidemiology. A report from the restless legs syndrome diagnosis and epidemiology workshop at the National Institutes of Health. *Sleep Med*. 2003;4:101-119.

25. Winkelman JW, Johnston L. Augmentation and tolerance with long-term pramipexole treatment of restless legs syndrome (RLS). *Sleep Med*. 2004;5:9-14.

26. Benes H, Heinrich CR, Ueberall MA, Kohnen R. Long-term safety and efficacy of cabergoline for the treatment of idiopathic restless legs syndrome: results from an open-label 6-month clinical trial. *Sleep*. 2004;27:674-682.

27. Stiasny-Kolster K, Benes H, Peglau I, et al. Effective cabergoline treatment in idiopathic restless legs syndrome. *Neurology*. 2004;63:2272-2279.

28. Silber MH, Shepard JW Jr, Wisbey JA. Pergolide in the management of restless legs syndrome: an extended study. *Sleep*. 1997;20:878-882.

29. Winkelmann J, Wetter TC, Stiasny K, Oertel WH, Trenkwalder C. Treatment of restless leg syndrome with pergolide--an open clinical trial. *Mov Disord*. 1998;13:566-569.

30. Earley CJ, Yaffee JB, Allen RP. Randomized, double-blind, placebo-controlled trial of pergolide in restless legs syndrome. *Neurology*. 1998;51:1599-1602.

31. Garcia-Borreguero D, Grunstein R, Sridhar G, et al. A 52-week open-label study of the long-term safety of ropinirole in patients with restless legs syndrome. *Sleep Med*. 2007;8(7-8):742-752.

32. Ondo W, Romanyshyn J, Vuong KD, Lai D. Long-term treatment of restless legs syndrome with dopamine agonists. *Arch Neurol*. 2004;61:1393-1397.

33. Kvernmo T, Hartter S, Burger E. A review of the receptor-binding and pharmacokinetic properties of dopamine agonists. *Clin Ther*. 2006;28:1065-1078.

34. Kains JP, Hardy JC, Chevalier C, Collier A. Retroperitoneal fibrosis in two patients with Parkinson's disease treated with bromocriptine. *Acta Clin Belg*. 1990;45:306-310.

35. Sanchez-Chapado M, Angulo Cuesta J, Guil Cid M, Jimenez FJ, Lopez Alvarez YJ. Retroperitoneal fibrosis secondary to treatment with L-dopa analogues for Parkinson disease. *Arch Esp Urol*. 1995;48:979-983.

36. Danoff SK, Grasso ME, Terry PB, Flynn JA. Pleuropulmonary disease due to pergolide use for restless legs syndrome. *Chest*. 2001;120:313-316.

37. Townsend M, MacIver DH. Constrictive pericarditis and pleuropulmonary fibrosis secondary to cabergoline treatment for Parkinson's disease. *Heart*. 2004;90:e47.

38. Champagne S, Coste E, Peyriere H, et al. Chronic constrictive pericarditis induced by long-term bromocriptine therapy: report of two cases. *Ann Pharmacother*. 1999;33:1050-1054.

39. Serratrice J, Disdier P, Habib G, Viallet F, Weiller PJ. Fibrotic valvular heart disease subsequent to bromocriptine treatment. *Cardiol Rev*. 2002;10:334-336.

40. Balachandran KP, Stewart D, Berg GA, Oldroyd KG. Chronic pericardial constriction linked to the antiparkinsonian dopamine agonist pergolide. *Postgrad Med J*. 2002;78:49-50.

41. Horvath J, Fross RD, Kleiner-Fisman G, et al. Severe multivalvular heart disease: a new complication of the ergot derivative dopamine agonists. *Mov Disord*. 2004;19:656-662.

42. Junghanns S, Fuhrmann JT, Simonis G, et al. Valvular heart disease in Parkinson's disease patients treated with dopamine agonists: a reader-blinded monocenter echocardiography study. *Mov Disord*. 2007;22:234-238.

43. Zanettini R, Antonini A, Gatto G, Gentile R, Tesei S, Pezzoli G. Valvular heart disease and the use of dopamine agonists for Parkinson's disease. *N Engl J Med*. 2007;356:39-46.

44. Horowski R, Jahnichen S, Pertz HH. Fibrotic valvular heart disease is not related to chemical class but to biological function: 5-HT2B receptor activation plays crucial role. *Mov Disord*. 2004;19:1523-1524.

45. Jahnichen S, Horowski R, Pertz HH. Agonism at 5-HT2B receptors is not a class effect of the ergolines. *Eur J Pharmacol*. 2005;513:225-228.

46. Hofmann C, Penner U, Dorow R, et al. Lisuride, a dopamine receptor agonist with 5-HT2B receptor antagonist properties: absence of cardiac valvulopathy adverse drug reaction reports supports the concept of a crucial role for 5-HT2B receptor agonism in cardiac valvular fibrosis. *Clin Neuropharmacol*. 2006;29:80-86.

47. Tribl GG, Sycha T, Kotzailias N, Zeitlhofer J, Auff E. Apomorphine in idiopathic restless legs syndrome: an exploratory study. *J Neurol Neurosurg Psychiatry*. 2005;76:181-185.

48. Reuter I, Ellis CM, Ray Chaudhuri K. Nocturnal subcutaneous apomorphine infusion in Parkinson's disease and restless legs syndrome. *Acta Neurol Scand*. 1999;100:163-167.

49. Tings T, Stiens G, Paulus W, Trenkwalder C, Happe S. Treatment of restless legs syndrome with subcutaneous apomorphine in a patient with short bowel syndrome. *J Neurol*. 2005;252:361-363.

50. Akpinar S. Restless legs syndrome treatment with dopaminergic drugs. *Clin Neuropharmacol*. 1987;10:69-79.

51. Walters AS, Hening WA, Kavey N, Chokroverty S, Gidro-Frank S. A double-blind randomized crossover trial of bromocriptine and placebo in restless legs syndrome. *Ann Neurol*. 1988;24:455-458.

52. Becker PM, Jamieson AO, Brown WD. Dopaminergic agents in restless legs syndrome and periodic limb movements of sleep: response and complications of extended treatment in 49 cases. *Sleep*. 1993;16:713-716.

53. Benes H, Heinrich CR, Ueberall MA, Kohnen R. Long-term safety and efficacy of cabergoline for the treatment of idiopathic restless legs syndrome: results from an open-label 6-month clinical trial. *Sleep*. 2004;27:674-682.

54. Stiasny-Kolster K, Benes H, Peglau I, et al. Effective cabergoline treatment in idiopathic restless legs syndrome. *Neurology*. 2004;63:2272-2279.

55. Trenkwalder C, Benes H, Grote L, et al; CALDIR Study Group. Cabergoline compared to levodopa in the treatment of patients with severe restless legs syndrome: results from a multi-center, randomized, active controlled trial. *Mov Disord*. 2007;22:696-703.

56. Benes H. Transdermal lisuride: short-term efficacy and tolerability study in patients with severe restless legs syndrome. *Sleep Med*. 2006;7:31-35.

57. Benes H, Deissler A, Rodenbeck A, Engfer A, Kohnen R. Lisuride treatment of restless legs syndrome: first studies with monotherapy in de novo patients and in combination with levodopa in advanced disease. *J Neural Transm*. 2006;113:87-92.

58. Silber MH, Shepard JW Jr, Wisbey JA. Pergolide in the management of restless legs syndrome: an extended study. *Sleep*. 1997;20:878-882.

59. Earley CJ, Yaffee JB, Allen RP. Randomized, double-blind, placebo-controlled trial of pergolide in restless legs syndrome. *Neurology*. 1998;51:1599-1602.

60. Stiasny K, Wetter TC, Winkelmann J, et al. Long-term effects of pergolide in the treatment of restless legs syndrome. *Neurology*. 2001;56:1399-1402.

61. Trenkwalder C, Hundemer HP, Lledo A, et al ; PEARLS Study Group. Efficacy of pergolide in treatment of restless legs syndrome: the PEARLS Study. *Neurology*. 2004;62:1391-1397.

62. Evidente VG. Piribedil for restless legs syndrome: a pilot study. *Mov Disord*. 2001;16:579-581.

63. Stiasny-Kolster K, Kohnen R, Schollmayer E, Moller JC, Oertel WH; Rotigotine Sp 666 Study Group. Patch application of the dopamine agonist rotigotine to patients with moderate to advanced stages of restless legs syndrome: a double-blind, placebo-controlled pilot study. *Mov Disord*. 2004;19:1432-1438.

64. Oertel WH, Benes H, Garcia-Borreguero D; On behalf of the Rotigotine SP 709 Study Group. Efficacy of rotigotine transdermal system in severe restless legs syndrome: A randomized, double-blind, placebo-controlled, six-week dose-finding trial in Europe. *Sleep Med*. 2007 June 4; Epub ahead of print.

65. Lapka R, Marek J, Rejholec V, Franc Z. Pharmacokinetics of oral terguride in patients with a prolactinoma. *Eur J Clin Pharmacol*. 1986;30:363-365.

66. Sonka K, Pretl M, Kranda K. Management of restless legs syndrome by the partial D2-agonist terguride. *Sleep Med*. 2003;4:455-457.

67. Lundvall O, Abom PE, Holm R. Carbamazepine in restless legs. A controlled pilot study. *Eur J Clin Pharmacol*. 1983;25:323-324.

68. Mellick GA, Mellick LB. Management of restless legs syndrome with gabapentin (Neurontin) *Sleep*. 1996;19:224-226.

69. Happe S, Klosch G, Saletu B, Zeitlhofer J. Treatment of idiopathic restless legs syndrome (RLS) with gabapentin. *Neurology*. 2001;57:1717-1719.

70. Garcia-Borreguero D, Larrosa O, de la Llave Y, Verger K, Masramon X, Hernandez G. Treatment of restless legs syndrome with gabapentin: a double-blind, cross-over study. *Neurology*. 2002;59:1573-1579.

71. Happe S, Sauter C, Klosch G, Saletu B, Zeitlhofer J. Gabapentin versus ropinirole in the treatment of idiopathic restless legs syndrome. *Neuropsychobiology*. 2003;48:82-86.

72. Thorp ML, Morris CD, Bagby SP. A crossover study of gabapentin in treatment of restless legs syndrome among hemodialysis patients. *Am J Kidney Dis*. 2001;38:104-108.

73. Micozkadioglu H, Ozdemir FN, Kut A, Sezer S, Saatci U, Haberal M. Gabapentin versus levodopa for the treatment of Restless Legs Syndrome in hemodialysis patients: an open-label study. *Ren Fail*. 2004;26:393-397.

74. Telstad W, Sorensen O, Larsen S, Lillevold PE, Stensrud P, Nyberg-Hansen R. Treatment of the restless legs syndrome with carbamazepine: a double blind study. *Br Med J* (Clin Res Ed). 1984;288:444-446.

189

75. Sorensen O, Telstad W. Carbamazepine (Tegretol) in restless legs. *Tidsskr Nor Laegeforen.* 1984;104:2093-2095.

76. Larsen S, Telstad W, Sorensen O, Thom E, Stensrud P, Nyberg-Hansen R. Carbamazepine therapy in restless legs. Discrimination between responders and non-responders. *Acta Med Scand.* 1985;218:223-227.

77. Youssef EA, Wagner ML, Martinez JO, Hening W. Pilot trial of lamotrigine in the restless legs syndrome. *Sleep Med.* 2005;6:89.

78. Della Marca G, Vollono C, Mariotti P, et al. Levetiracetam can be effective in the treatment of restless legs syndrome with periodic limb movements in sleep: report of two cases. *J Neurol Neurosurg Psychiatry.* 2006;77:566-567.

79. Ozturk O, Eraslan D, Kumral E. Oxcarbazepine treatment for paroxetine-induced restless leg syndrome. *Gen Hosp Psychiatry.* 2006;28:264-265.

80. Sommer M, Bachmann CG, Liebetanz KM, Schindehutte J, Tings T, Paulus W. Pregabalin in restless legs syndrome with and without neuropathic pain. *Acta Neurol Scand.* 2007;115:347-350.

81. Perez Bravo A. Topiramate use as treatment in restless legs syndrome. *Actas Esp Psiquiatr.* 2004;32:132-137.

82. Eisensehr I, Ehrenberg BL, Rogge Solti S, Noachtar S. Treatment of idiopathic restless legs syndrome (RLS) with slow-release valproic acid compared with slow-release levodopa/benserazid. *J Neurol.* 2004;251:579-583.

83. Ekbom KA. Restless legs syndrome. *Neurology.* 1960;10:868-873.

84. Trzepacz PT, Violette EJ, Sateia MJ. Response to opioids in three patients with restless legs syndrome. *Am J Psychiatry.* 1984;141:993-995.

85. Walters A, Hening W, Cote L, Fahn S. Dominantly inherited restless legs with myoclonus and periodic movements of sleep: a syndrome related to the endogenous opiates? *Adv Neurol.* 1986;43:309-19.

86. Sandyk R, Gillman MA. The opioid system in the restless legs and nocturnal myoclonus syndromes. *Sleep.* 1986;9:370-371.

87. Hening WA, Walters A, Kavey N, Gidro-Frank S, Cote L, Fahn S. Dyskinesias while awake and periodic movements in sleep in restless legs syndrome: treatment with opioids. *Neurology.* 1986;36:1363-1366.

88. Winkelmann J, Schadrack J, Wetter TC, Zieglgansberger W, Trenkwalder C. Opioid and dopamine antagonist drug challenges in untreated restless legs syndrome patients. *Sleep Med.* 2001;2:57-61.

89. Walters AS. Review of receptor agonist and antagonist studies relevant to the opiate system in restless legs syndrome. *Sleep Med.* 2002;3:301-304.

90. Montplaisir J, Lorrain D, Godbout R. Restless legs syndrome and periodic leg movements in sleep: the primary role of dopaminergic mechanism. *Eur Neurol*. 1991;31:41-43.

91. Walters AS, Winkelmann J, Trenkwalder C, et al. Long-term follow-up on restless legs syndrome patients treated with opioids. *Mov Disord*. 2001;16:1105-1109.

92. Dayer P, Collart L, Desmeules J. The pharmacology of tramadol. *Drugs*. 1994;47(suppl 1):3-7.

93. Preston KL, Jasinski DR, Testa M. Abuse potential and pharmacological comparison of tramadol and morphine. *Drug Alcohol Depend*. 1991;27:7-17.

94. Cicero TJ, Inciardi JA, Adams EH, et al. Rates of abuse of tramadol remain unchanged with the introduction of new branded and generic products: results of an abuse monitoring system, 1994-2004. *Pharmacoepidemiol Drug Saf*. 2005;14:851-859.

95. Adams EH, Breiner S, Cicero TJ, et al. A comparison of the abuse liability of tramadol, NSAIDs, and hydrocodone in patients with chronic pain. *J Pain Symptom Manage*. 2006;31:465-476.

96. Lauerma H, Markkula J. Treatment of restless legs syndrome with tramadol: an open study. *J Clin Psychiatry*. 1999;60:241-244.

97. Ondo WG. Methadone for refractory restless legs syndrome. *Mov Disord*. 2005;20:345-348.

98. Davis MP, Walsh D. Methadone for relief of cancer pain: a review of pharmacokinetics, pharmacodynamics, drug interactions and protocols of administration. *Support Care Cancer*. 2001;9:73-83.

99. Sees KL, Delucchi KL, Masson C, et al. Methadone maintenance vs 180-day psychosocially enriched detoxification for treatment of opioid dependence: a randomized controlled trial. *JAMA*. 2000;283:1303-1310.

100. Blake AD, Bot G, Freeman JC, Reisine T. Differential opioid agonist regulation of the mouse mu opioid receptor. *J Biol Chem*. 1997;272:782-790.

101. Jakobsson B, Ruuth K. Successful treatment of restless legs syndrome with an implanted pump for intrathecal drug delivery. *Acta Anaesthesiol Scand*. 2002;46:114-117.

102. Vahedi H, Kuchle M, Trenkwalder C, Krenz CJ. Peridural morphine administration in restless legs status. *Anasthesiol Intensivmed Notfallmed Schmerzther*. 1994;29:368-370.

103. Walters AS, Wagner ML, Hening WA, et al. Successful treatment of the idiopathic restless legs syndrome in a randomized double-blind trial of oxycodone versus placebo. *Sleep*. 1993;16:327-332.

104. Matthews WB. Treatment of the restless legs syndrome with clonazepam. *Br Med J*. 1979;1:751.

9

105. Allen RP, Picchietti D, Hening WA, Trenkwalder C, Walters AS, Montplaisi J; Restless Legs Syndrome Diagnosis and Epidemiology workshop at the National Institutes of Health; International Restless Legs Syndrome Study Group. Restless legs syndrome: diagnostic criteria, special considerations, and epidemiology. A report from the restless legs syndrome diagnosis and epidemiology workshop at the National Institutes of Health. *Sleep Med.* 2003;4:101-119.

106. Allen RP, Lesage S, Earley CJ. Anti-histamines and benzodiazepines exacerbate daytime restless legs syndrome (RLS) symptoms. *Sleep.* 2005;28:A279. Abstract.

107. Mitler MM, Browman CP, Menn SJ, Gujavarty K, Timms RM. Nocturnal myoclonus: treatment efficacy of clonazepam and temazepam. *Sleep.* 1986;9:385-392.

108. Scharf MB, Brown L, Hirschowitz J. Possible efficacy of alprazolam in restless leg syndrome. *Hillside J Clin Psychiatry.* 1986;8:214-223.

109. Boghen D. Successful treatment of restless legs with clonazepam. *Ann Neurol.* 1980;8:341.

110. Montagna P, Sassoli de Bianchi L, Zucconi M, Cirignotta F, Lugaresi E. Clonazepam and vibration in restless legs syndrome. *Acta Neurol Scand.* 1984;69:428-430.

111. Boghen D, Lamothe L, Elie R, Godbout R, Montplasir J. The treatment of the restless legs syndrome with clonazepam: a prospective controlled study. *Can J Neurol Sci.* 1986;13:245-247.

112. Tollefson G, Erdman C. Triazolam in the restless legs syndrome. *J Clin Psychopharmacol.* 1985;5:361-362.

113. Doghramji K, Browman CP, Gaddy JR, Walsh JK. Triazolam diminishes daytime sleepiness and sleep fragmentation in patients with periodic leg movements in sleep. *J Clin Psychopharmacol.* 1991;11:284-290.

114. Bonnet MH, Arand DL. Chronic use of triazolam in patients with periodic leg movements, fragmented sleep and daytime sleepiness. *Aging* (Milano). 1991;3:313-324.

115. Borja NL, Daniel KL. Ramelteon for the treatment of insomnia. *Clin Ther.* 2006;28:1540-1555.

116. Bezerra ML, Martinez JV. Zolpidem in restless legs syndrome. *Eur Neurol.* 2002;48:180-181.

117. Morgenthaler TI, Silber MH. Amnestic sleep-related eating disorder associated with zolpidem. *Sleep Med.* 2002;3:323-327.

118. Evidente VG, Adler CH, Caviness JN, Hentz JG, Gwinn-Hardy K. Amantadine is beneficial in restless legs syndrome. *Mov Disord.* 2000;15:324-327.

119. Rotenberg JS, Canard K, Difazio M. Successful treatment of recalcitrant restless legs syndrome with botulinum toxin type-A. *J Clin Sleep Med.* 2006;2:275-278.

120. Handwerker JV Jr, Palmer RF. Clonidine in the treatment of "restless leg" syndrome. *N Engl J Med.* 1985;313:1228-1229.

121. Cavatorta F, Vagge R, Solari P, Queirolo C. Preliminary results with clonidine in the restless legs syndrome in 2 hemodialyzed uremic patients. *Minerva Urol Nefrol.* 1987;39:93.

122. Bastani B, Westervelt FB. Effectiveness of clonidine in alleviating the symptoms of "restless legs". *Am J Kidney Dis.* 1987;10:326.

123. Zoe A, Wagner ML, Walters AS. High-dose clonidine in a case of restless legs syndrome. *Ann Pharmacother.* 1994;28:878-881.

124. Wagner ML, Walters AS, Coleman RG, Hening WA, Grasing K, Chokroverty S. Randomized, double-blind, placebo-controlled study of clonidine in restless legs syndrome. *Sleep.* 1996;19:52-58.

125. Bamford CR, Sandyk R. Failure of clonidine to ameliorate the symptoms of restless legs syndrome. *Sleep.* 1987;10:398-399.

126. Strang RR. The symptom of restless legs. *Med J Aust.* 1967;1:1211-1213.

127. Lipinski JF, Zubenko GS, Barreira P, Cohen BM. Propranolol in the treatment of neuroleptic-induced akathisia. *Lancet.* 1983;2:685-686.

128. Derom E, Elinck W, Buylaert W, van der Straeten M. Which beta-blocker for the restless leg? *Lancet.* 1984;1:857.

129. Ginsberg HN. Propranolol in the treatment of restless legs syndrome induced by imipramine withdrawal. *Am J Psychiatry.* 1986;143:938.

130. O'Sullivan RL, Greenberg DB. H2 antagonists, restless leg syndrome, and movement disorders. *Psychosomatics.* 1993;34:530-532.

131. Botez MI. Folate deficiency and neurological disorders in adults. *Med Hypotheses.* 1976;2:135-140.

132. Botez MI, Cadotte M, Beaulieu R, Pichette LP, Pison C. Neurologic disorders responsive to folic acid therapy. *Can Med Assoc J.* 1976;115:217-223.

133. Ayres S Jr, Mihan R. Leg cramps (systremma) and "restless legs" syndrome. Response to vitamin E (tocopherol). *Calif Med.* 1969;111:87-91.

134. Ayres S Jr, Mihan R. Restless legs syndrome: response to vitamin E. *J Appl Nutr* 1973;25:8-15.

135. Botez MI, Fontaine F, Botez T, Bachevalier J. Folate-responsive neurological and mental disorders: report of 16 cases. Neuropsychological correlates of computerized transaxial tomography and radionuclide cisternography in folic acid deficiencies. *Eur Neurol.* 1977;16:230-246.

136. Lee KA, Zaffke ME, Baratte-Beebe K. Restless legs syndrome and sleep disturbance during pregnancy: the role of folate and iron. *J Womens Health Gend Based Med.* 2001;10:335-341.

9

137. Bateman PP. The "restless legs" syndrome. *Med J Aust.* 1991;155:135.

138. Hornyak M, Voderholzer U, Hohagen F, Berger M, Riemann D. Magnesium therapy for periodic leg movements-related insomnia and restless legs syndrome: an open pilot study. *Sleep.* 1998;21:501-505.

139. Walters AS, Elin RJ, Cohen B, Moller JC, Oertel W, Stiasny-Kolster K. Magnesium not likely to play a major role in the pathogenesis of Restless Legs Syndrome: serum and cerebrospinal fluid studies. *Sleep Med.* 2007;8:186-187.

140. Banerji NK, Hurwitz LJ. Restless legs syndrome, with particular reference to its occurrence after gastric surgery. *Br Med J.* 1970;4:774-775.

141. Hanna PA, Kumar S, Walters AS. Restless legs symptoms in a patient with above knee amputations: a case of phantom restless legs. *Clin Neuropharmacol.* 2004;27:87-89.

142. Cortese S, Konofal E, Lecendreux M, Mouren MC, Bernardina BD. Restless legs syndrome triggered by heart surgery. *Pediatr Neurol.* 2006;35:223-226.

143. Minai OA, Golish JA, Yataco JC, Budev MM, Blazey H, Giannini C. Restless legs syndrome in lung transplant recipients. *J Heart Lung Transplant.* 2007;26:24-29.

144. Walters AS, Wagner M, Hening WA. Periodic limb movements as the initial manifestation of restless legs syndrome triggered by lumbosacral radiculopathy. *Sleep.* 1996;19:825-826.

145. Yasuda T, Nishimura A, Katsuki Y, Tsuji Y. Restless legs syndrome treated successfully by kidney transplantation—a case report. *Clin Transpl.* 1986:138.

146. Winkelmann J, Stautner A, Samtleben W, Trenkwalder C. Long-term course of restless legs syndrome in dialysis patients after kidney transplantation. *Mov Disord.* 2002;17:1072-1076.

147. Rye DB, DeLong MR. Amelioration of sensory limb discomfort of restless legs syndrome by pallidotomy. *Ann Neurol.* 1999;46:800-801.

148. Driver-Dunckley E, Evidente VG, Adler CH, et al. Restless legs syndrome in Parkinson's disease patients may improve with subthalamic stimulation. *Mov Disord.* 2006;21:1287-1289.

149. Ondo W. VIM deep brain stimulation does not improve pre-existing restless legs syndrome in patients with essential tremor. *Parkinsonism Relat Disord.* 2006;12:113-114.

10

Approaching the Patient With RLS

Although people with restless legs syndrome (RLS) may seem symptomatically quite similar at first, they are actually a diverse group of patients who often present with different needs for treatment. To help decide on the most appropriate of the available therapies, several algorithms have been constructed to help guide physicians to a practical approach to treating RLS patients.[1-7]

A number of these algorithms categorize the treatment based on the frequency of symptoms, which tends to be an effective starting point. Suggestions from most of these articles are considered in this chapter, but the treatment recommendation is patterned most closely on the algorithms discussed in the more recent articles. These algorithms are further augmented with practical suggestions based on considerable clinical experience.

Patients With Intermittent Symptoms

Intermittent RLS is defined as RLS that is troublesome enough when present to require treatment but does not occur frequently enough to necessitate daily therapy. People with intermittent symptoms represent the largest group of those with RLS. They embody a wide spectrum of the disease with symptoms that may occur once every few months to a few times per week. As such, they often need somewhat different therapy based on the frequency, time of day, and intensity of symptoms.

In general, people with intermittent RLS tend to have milder symptoms and respond more readily to treatment than those with daily symptoms. Therefore, this group of patients is usually easier to treat. However, as they are still quite a diverse group, treatment should be individualized as discussed below.

The general approach to treating these patients is detailed in the algorithm for the management of intermittent RLS in **Figure 10.1**. Often, the RLS symptoms may respond to nonpharmacologic therapies (see Chapter 8, *Nonpharmacologic Management/Lifestyle Modifications*) and totally avoid the need for drugs. However, even if these nondrug therapies are successful, there may still be occasions when these techniques are not adequate and medication may be necessary. It is often wise to prescribe as-needed (prn) medication for sporadic use when the nondrug therapies are not sufficient. Similar medications can be chosen to those for patients who rely on medications to relieve their symptoms (**Table 10.1**).

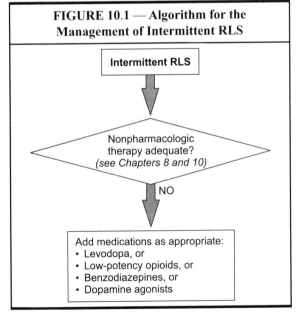

FIGURE 10.1 — Algorithm for the Management of Intermittent RLS

Intermittent RLS

Nonpharmacologic therapy adequate? *(see Chapters 8 and 10)*

NO

Add medications as appropriate:
• Levodopa, or
• Low-potency opioids, or
• Benzodiazepines, or
• Dopamine agonists

TABLE 10.1 — Drugs for Intermittent RLS	
Type of RLS Problem	**Suitable Drugs**
Bedtime RLS	
Infrequent	Sedative/hypnotics, opioid analgesics, or L-dopa
≥3 nights/week	Approved dopamine agonists agonists
Daytime RLS	
Expected	Dopamine agonists, L-dopa, opioid analgesics
Unexpected	Opioid analgesics or L-dopa
One drug fits all needs	Opioid analgesics or L-dopa

■ Instituting Nonpharmacologic Therapy
Avoid Medications That Worsen RLS

Physicians should start by reviewing the patient's medication list, including medications that are taken on an as-needed basis and over-the-counter ones. When possible, drugs that worsen RLS should be changed to more RLS-friendly ones (*Chapter 8* and Chapter 12, *RLS and Psychiatric Disorders*). Patients should be advised to obtain an RLS medical-alert card so that they can be aware of these medications and can also warn their other physicians who may not be as knowledgeable about the disorder.

Abstinence from Alcohol, Caffeine, and Nicotine

There should be a review of dietary and other habits to help eliminate alcohol, caffeine, and nicotine. Counseling and other treatments may be necessary to help patients avoid these often-addicting behaviors.

Develop a "Bag of Tricks"

Patients should be advised to plan for situations that worsen RLS. For example, alerting activities may be helpful for sedentary situations (eg, airplane trips) that typically trigger RLS. They may need to bring a deck of cards, hand-held video game, crossword puzzle, or other mentally engaging activities when going on trips. However, many other activities (eg, stretches, exercises, hot or cold baths, and other counterstimulation activities) may help RLS. Patients should be advised to develop a large bag of tricks that contains a variety of techniques to help cope with all of the diverse situations that may trigger or worsen RLS.

Sleep Hygiene

Proper sleep hygiene is often essential for RLS patients to minimize their symptoms. As with insomnia, which occurs frequently in RLS patients, it is important to review the rules of sleep hygiene (discussed in *Chapter 8*) and assure that patients are getting adequate sleep.

Exercise

Mild-to-moderate levels of exercise have been demonstrated to improve RLS symptoms.[8] Patients should be counseled to perform regular (at least three to four times per week) exercise that may help their RLS and provide other health benefits.

Education and Support Groups

RLS patients should be encouraged to join the RLS Foundation (*www.rls.org*), and if available, a local support group. This involvement helps patients become educated about RLS and learn how to live with their disease. Speaking with other RLS patients often gives them insights on dealing with friends, family, and coworkers and may be an invaluable source for adding to their bag of tricks. In addition, there are many websites with information on RLS as well as forums and chat groups that can benefit RLS patients (see *Appendix B*).

Iron Therapy

RLS patients should have their serum ferritin level determined even when their hemoglobin and serum iron levels are normal. The serum ferritin level is the most accurate and sensitive test (other than a bone marrow evaluation) to determine whether iron stores are low. Serum ferritin levels <50 ug/mL (despite lab-reported normal levels of >10-20 ug/mL) have been associated with an increased severity of RLS,[9,10] and treating these patients with supplemental iron may help their RLS. For further discussion on the administration of iron therapy for RLS, see Secondary RLS in Chapter 11, *Special Considerations*.

■ Instituting Drug Therapy for Intermittent RLS

Even patients with mild, infrequent RLS symptoms have occasions when the nondrug therapies discussed are not sufficient and medication may be needed. Their RLS may be exacerbated by a long airplane trip, medication, anxiety, or many other various triggers. As noted, it is helpful to prescribe as-needed medication for most RLS patients.

As of now, no medications are approved for intermittent use as treatment of RLS and studies of intermittent RLS are rare. However, expert opinion based on significant clinical experience can provide some suggestions for managing these patients. Medications for those with intermittent RLS can be chosen from the algorithm in **Figure 10.1** and guided by **Table 10.1**. The choice of medication should match the frequency and timing of the symptoms. For example, it is clear that a sedative hypnotic drug may be appropriate for bedtime RLS but not for daytime symptoms.

Infrequent Bedtime RLS

Bedtime presents significant problems for most RLS sufferers. Symptoms tend to be peaking and effective treatment should be instituted promptly to avoid increased anxiety that may further hamper sleep. Therefore, a quick-acting agent is the most appropriate choice in this situation.

Which of the drugs listed in **Table 10**.1 for infrequent bedtime RLS is the best choice for this situation? They are all reasonable choices and it depends more upon how well the drug works for the individual patient and the comfort level the physician has concerning prescribing them.

Any of the sedative hypnotic drugs are suitable for bedtime RLS symptoms; the onset of most of them is rapid and they typically accomplish the main goal of enabling the patient to fall asleep. As per the discussion of these drugs in Chapter 9, *Medications and Other Medical Treatments*, hypnotics with a shorter half-life are a better choice, although if sleep maintenance is a concern, drugs with a somewhat longer half-life may be warranted. There is also less concern about tolerance and dependence when using these drugs on an intermittent basis.

Opioid analgesics, which include the opioids and tramadol (see *Chapter 9*) are also effective for treating bedtime RLS. They tend to onset quickly and are potent for relieving RLS symptoms. As with the sedative hypnotics, there is less concern about tolerance and dependence when using them intermittently. Typically, the low-potency opioids (most clinicians use propoxyphene or codeine) are used but smaller doses of the medium-potency drugs may be equally appropriate (½ of a hydrocodone or tramadol tablet).

L-dopa containing drugs (carbidopa/L-dopa or benserazide/L-dopa) are also good choices in this situation. These drugs have a quick onset, typically within 30 minutes or as fast as 15 minutes on an empty stomach. There is no concern about augmentation with L-dopa when used on an intermittent basis.

Frequent Bedtime RLS

The choice of ≥3 days per week to define frequent RLS is arbitrary. However, bedtime symptoms that occur at a similar frequency and significantly decrease sleep time can be disruptive enough to warrant daily therapy. Although it may still be appropriate to use the medications listed for infrequent bedtime RLS, it may be better to avoid these symptoms completely by prophylactically treating them daily with an approved dopamine agonist taken 1 to 3 hours before bedtime.

If the RLS symptoms are frequent but milder and do not always significantly disturb sleep, the drugs suggested for infrequent RLS may be appropriate. Each patient should be considered individually and a treatment plan that fits his or her needs should be devised using the described guidelines.

Expected Daytime RLS

Many people with intermittent RLS can easily predict when their RLS will typically worsen and require drug treatment for such situations. Common examples are evening movies or airplane trips. Patients can plan to take medication before symptoms occur. This is generally a good idea as it avoids any suffering and lower doses are often effective when taken prior to the onset of symptoms.

The dopamine agonists are a reasonable choice for this situation as they can be taken 1 to 3 hours prior to the provocation and, due to their long half-life, can protect patients for prolonged situations, such as airplane or other trips. Some patients may prefer to wait and see if symptoms occur or can be eliminated with nondrug therapy. For those, the quicker-acting opioid analgesics (low-potency opioids or tramadol) and L-dopa may be reasonable. These drugs can also be used prophylactically before situations of shorter duration that exacerbate RLS. Analgesic drugs may cause daytime sedation and, therefore, may be inappropriate for some individuals and for activities that require alertness, such as theater or other public entertainment.

The best drug for this situation is the one that the patient tolerates, is effective, and fits their needs. In some cases, it may take trial and error to determine the proper choice of therapy.

Unexpected Daytime RLS

Despite the best planning and intentions, there will be situations that occur when patients forget to take their medications prophylactically or symptoms just appear at unexpected times. This situation is similar to infrequent bedtime RLS in that quick relief is necessary. Therefore, the choice of drug is also similar, except that the sedative hypnotic drugs are usually inappropriate, as alertness is impaired. An exception may be a long airplane flight. However, if the person is awakened in flight (eg, when served a meal), RLS symptoms may promptly return.

Therefore, the choice is usually between the opioid analgesics (low-potency opioids or tramadol) and L-dopa. Again, the correct drug is the one that is best tolerated, most effective, and fits the patient's needs.

One Drug Fits All Needs

Many patients may fit into one of the described categories, but commonly patients may have multiple needs. RLS symptoms may appear unpredictably at odd times and cause both bedtime and daytime problems. Physicians may also need to treat exacerbations that are more predictable.

Although some patients may prefer to have an arsenal of medications to treat their RLS in all of the different potential situations, it may be simpler to prescribe one medication that can be used in all the described situations. Opioid analgesics and L-dopa fit most of these needs fairly well. Either of these drugs is a good choice for patients who have intermittent RLS that does not warrant regular medication. These medications are also good choices for as-needed use in patients who need daily medication and in those who rely on nondrug therapy but may need medication on rare occasions. The latter group of patients may be thankful to have medication available for those unusual times when nothing else works.

Patients With Daily RLS

Daily RLS is defined as RLS that is frequent and troublesome enough to require daily therapy (**Figure 10.2**). Despite employing all of the beneficial non-pharmacologic therapies, patients with this condition continue to suffer from symptoms that require daily treatment with drugs.

Dopamine agonists are considered the drugs of choice for daily RLS and are the only FDA- and European-approved medications (pramipexole and ropinirole).[11-15] Therefore, unless there is a contraindication, physicians should start treatment of patients with daily RLS symptoms with one of these dopamine agonists. These drugs should be started at their lowest dose and titrated slowly until symptoms are relieved as per the guidelines in *Chapter 9*.

Alternatively, as per **Figure 10.2**, non-approved dopamine agonists, gabapentin (or other anticonvulsants) or low-potency opioids, may be prescribed if treatment with the approved dopamine agonists is contraindicated or unsuccessful. Patients with painful RLS symptoms, an associated painful peripheral neuropathy, other unrelated chronic pain syndrome, or RLS in association with neurodegenerative disorders (eg, Parkinson's disease or dementia), are appropriate candidates for the anticonvulsants. As noted in *Chapter 9,* sedation often limits the use of these drugs, especially when given for daytime symptoms.

10

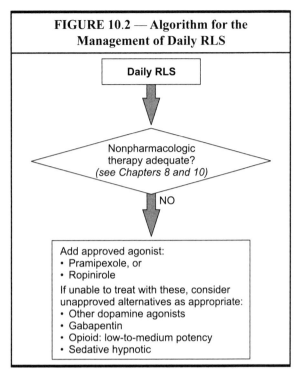

FIGURE 10.2 — Algorithm for the Management of Daily RLS

Daily RLS

Nonpharmacologic therapy adequate?
(see Chapters 8 and 10)

NO

Add approved agonist:
• Pramipexole, or
• Ropinirole

If unable to treat with these, consider unapproved alternatives as appropriate:
• Other dopamine agonists
• Gabapentin
• Opioid: low-to-medium potency
• Sedative hypnotic

The low-potency opioids may be suitable for some RLS patients, as they tend to be well tolerated, are inexpensive, and have a quick onset. Lower doses of the medium-potency opioids or tramadol can also be considered, as their effects are reasonably similar and are safe for long-term use (however, their use should be monitored closely to avoid tolerance and dependence occurring).

Both the anticonvulsants and opioids should be used at their lowest effective doses as per the guidelines discussed in *Chapter 9.*

Patients With Refractory RLS

Refractory RLS is defined as daily RLS treated with one or more dopamine agonist with one or more of the following outcomes:

- Inadequate initial response despite adequate doses
- Response that has become inadequate with time, despite increasing doses
- Intolerable adverse effects
- Augmentation that is not controllable with additional earlier doses of the drug.

These patients include the most difficult to manage RLS patients. Since few studies have been performed to determine how these patients should be treated, the recommendations in this section are based on the considerable experience of experts in the field. No drugs have been approved for patients who cannot be managed with the approved dopamine agonists and no drugs are approved to be used in combination with the approved dopamine agonists. While there is no single, recognized means of managing these patients, **Figure 10**.3 provides a general schema that illustrates some of the useful therapeutic strategies that have worked for those experienced with managing these patients. As primary care physicians become more familiar with RLS, they should be able to care for many of these patients, especially with the aid of this section. However, referral to an RLS specialist may be an appropriate option when patients are not responding to treatment as expected.

Each of the situations resulting in refractory RLS will be discussed and specific suggestions provided for them. Following the suggestions should aid physicians to treat a significant number of these more difficult RLS patients.

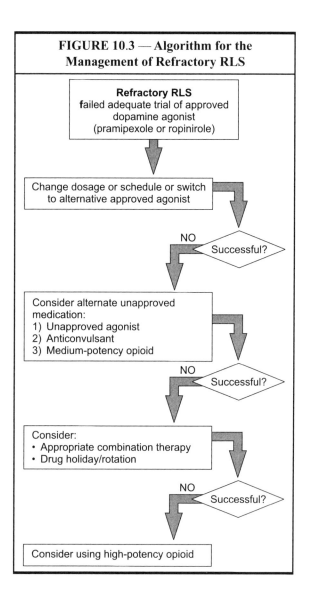

FIGURE 10.3 — Algorithm for the Management of Refractory RLS

Refractory RLS
failed adequate trial of approved dopamine agonist (pramipexole or ropinirole)

↓

Change dosage or schedule or switch to alternative approved agonist

Successful? — NO

Consider alternate unapproved medication:
1) Unapproved agonist
2) Anticonvulsant
3) Medium-potency opioid

Successful? — NO

Consider:
• Appropriate combination therapy
• Drug holiday/rotation

Successful? — NO

Consider using high-potency opioid

■ Inadequate Initial Response Despite Adequate Doses

As discussed, dopamine agonists should be started at the lowest available dose then increased slowly until symptoms are relieved. Since >90% of RLS patients respond to dopaminergic drugs,[16] only a small percentage will fall into the category of refractory RLS. Although some patients seem to respond only to high doses of these drugs, most do well with the lower dose ranges tabulated in **Table 9**.**3**. Physicians should be careful in exceeding the typical dose ranges of dopaminergics, as further titration will probably result in more side effects than relief.

Once reasonable doses of the drug have proved ineffective, other strategies need to be considered. Often, if one dopamine agonist lacks efficacy, another one may work better. Patients clearly differ in their responses to these drugs, so if one does not help, another should be tried before giving up on this class.

If dopamine agonists provide no relief, it is best to change to another class of drug. Gabapentin (or other anticonvulsants) and high-potency opioids are the next choices (**Figure 10**.**3**). Either of these drugs is a reasonable choice but typically the more severe RLS cases that comprise refractory patients respond better to the potent opioids. As discussed in *Chapter 9*, opioids should not be withheld from these patients, as they are very effective and safe when monitored and used according to the dosing guidelines in **Table 9**.**7**. In patients without a history of drug abuse, dependence, tolerance, or addiction is very unusual.

If the dopamine agonist helps somewhat but does not completely relieve all of the RLS symptoms, adding an additional medication is often beneficial. Sedative hypnotics may be helpful for bedtime RLS that does not fully respond to dopamine drugs. The addition of gabapentin (or other anticonvulsants) may relieve painful symptoms. If these strategies are not

207

sufficient, opioids can be added as needed. At times, all of these classes of drugs may be necessary to provide relief (see following section on combination therapy).

■ Response That Has Become Inadequate With Time Despite Increasing Doses

Many patients initially respond well to dopamine agonists. However, after time (typically many months to years), this response may wane. Whether this is due to worsening of RLS by a new trigger, tolerance to the drug, or the natural progression of the disease is often difficult to discern. Regardless of the etiology, this can be a difficult problem to solve.

Similar to the suggestions for an inadequate initial response to a dopamine agonist, care should be taken not to exceed the recommended dose ranges before deciding that alternative treatment is necessary.

Worsening Due to a New Trigger

It is not uncommon for RLS patients to be prescribed medications that worsen RLS, such as antidepressants. Therefore, when patients present with a diminished response to therapy, it is always worthwhile to review their complete medication list (both prescription and over the counter) thoroughly. Often changes can be made that are more RLS friendly and still treat the comorbid problem (see *Chapter 8* and *Chapter 12* for suggestions).

This is often an appropriate time to reassess the patient's serum ferritin level. As iron levels can diminish slowly, this problem may occur unexpectedly and respond to iron therapy.

Worsening Due to Tolerance

It is always possible that tolerance to the dopamine agonist may have developed with time. Usually, an increase in the dose will overcome this problem. However, when doses exceed the recommended ranges, other strategies should be considered. Typically, there is no cross-tolerance among dopamine agonists, so simply changing to another medication in this class should resolve the problem.

Sometimes tolerance develops within months to the second dopamine agonist. Often, changing to another dopamine agonist or even back to the original one may resolve this issue permanently or at least for several months. Some patients find benefit from rotating two or more dopamine agonists every few months (see the following section on rotating treatment).

If the aforementioned techniques do not help, following the algorithm's guidelines as discussed should provide relief.

Worsening Due to Progression of the Disease

RLS tends to be a slowly progressive disease with symptoms worsening over years to decades.[17] Although most patients continue to benefit from small increases in their dopamine agonist medication with this disease progression, some may experience more profound worsening of their symptoms that no longer respond to their dopamine agonist.

Once typical dose ranges are exceeded, the steps as outlined should be followed. These include a change to another dopamine agonist, to gabapentin or a opioid analgesic, or combination therapy.

■ Intolerable Side Effects

The dopamine agonists are typically well tolerated, especially at the lower doses used by RLS patients. However, some patients are sensitive to these drugs and will have trouble tolerating them. The most common side effect of the dopamine agonists is nausea, which may often be mitigated by taking the medication with food. Dizziness and postural hypotension may also occur, especially with the concomitant use of hypertensive medication or if patients become dehydrated.

209

In Europe and in Canada, domperidone (10 mg before doses or up to three times a day), a selective peripheral dopamine blocker, can be used to mitigate most side effects. (Americans may be able to obtain a supply from abroad.)

Sleepiness may actually be a beneficial side effect when the medication is taken at bedtime. However, if the drowsiness persists into the morning or if the medication is needed during the daytime, this problem may become disabling. Insomnia is another common side effect that may lead to discontinuation of the medication. If the problem is mild and can be resolved with occasional use of hypnotics, the dopamine agonist can be continued.

If any of the more serious but much less common side effects occur (eg, hallucinations, compulsive behavior, or paradoxic worsening of RLS), the medication must be stopped and other treatments instituted as per **Figure 10.3**.

■ Augmentation That Is Not Controllable With Additional Earlier Doses of the Drug

Augmentation (see *Chapter 9*) with dopamine agonists may be a mild problem that can treated simply by taking the drug earlier or adding an extra dose earlier in the day.[18,19] However, some patients progress quickly to needing medication very early in the day with a marked increase in the intensity of their symptoms. They often cannot sit for very long due to the increase in RLS symptoms, and increasing the dose of their dopaminergic drug only temporarily relieves the problem.

When RLS continues to worsen despite an escalation in the dopamine agonist dose, it is time to stop the medication and change therapy. Typically, medium- to high-potency opioids can be used to treat the marked exacerbation of RLS symptoms that occurs upon withdrawal of the drug. After several weeks, another dopamine agonist may be substituted and kept at a low dose. It is thought that longer-acting dopamine agonists (eg, cabergoline, rotigotine patch) may cause fewer problems with augmentation, but it is also possible that their long duration of action just treats the symptoms of augmentation.

If augmentation recurs with the new dopamine agonist, other treatment as outlined above and in **Figure 10.3** is indicated.

Individualized Treatment, Combination Treatment, Drug Holidays, and Rotating Treatment

■ **Individualized Treatment**

It would be nice if we could classify every patient into one of the treatment categories defined in this chapter. However, patients tend to have unique needs and problems that often are not solved by the recommendations in the described therapeutic plans. One of the keys to treating RLS patients is to be flexible. Often several different drugs, doses, and combinations need to be tried. At times, it may be quite frustrating to deal with this condition. However, with patience and guided trial and error, most RLS sufferers can achieve relief from even very bothersome symptoms.

Therapy with just one drug usually works well for most patients with mild-to-moderate RLS. However, many may still have special situations that require additional or different therapy as discussed below in combination therapy. For difficult cases, also consider drug holidays and rotating drugs.

Remember to treat daytime RLS symptoms. If they occur daily, then one or two extra doses of a dopamine agonist may be necessary. Add a quick-acting medication, such as L-dopa or an opioid analgesic, for as-needed use if daytime symptoms occur sporadically.

■ Combination Treatment

Patients with severe RLS tend to be more difficult to treat. Dopamine agonists alone often do not resolve their symptoms. Combining different classes of medication is frequently the key to treating RLS successfully. Furthermore, for patients who are sensitive to the side effects of medications, combination therapy allows for lower doses of each medication, which may decrease adverse reactions.

Adding a hypnotic for sleep can be helpful for many RLS patients as they often suffer from insomnia. Even those with mild intermittent RLS may have insomnia and benefit from such medication. An anticonvulsant to help decrease painful symptoms can also be helpful. By themselves, anticonvulsants usually are not as potent as the dopamine agonists or opioid analgesics for relieving RLS symptoms, but they may work well in combination with other drugs. However, it is often necessary to add an opioid to get control of the symptoms in patients with very severe and refractory disease. As discussed earlier in the section on refractory RLS, opioids should not be withheld when needed.

If symptoms are still not resolved after adding or trying all of the traditionally accepted RLS drugs earlier, think about adding a drug from the other RLS drug list. Being flexible may help solve difficult-to-treat RLS cases.

Milder cases also benefit from combination therapy. Although most of these patients do well with a daily evening dose of a dopamine agonist, many situations require additional therapy. Unexpected sedentary situations (ie, a movie or a trip), unexpected acute exacerbations of RLS, or just forgetting to take the medication on time all require quick treatment. Since the dopamine agonists require 1 to 3 hours until onset, a short-acting drug should be given to most patients for acute treatment. Typically, an opioid analgesic or L-dopa works best in these situations. Therefore, RLS patients should have a prescription for an opioid analgesic or L-dopa and keep a small supply in their car, purse, office, or other places where they can be easily accessed when needed.

■ **Drug Holidays**

The concept of drug holidays is associated with medications that may cause tolerance. Although the mechanism of tolerance is not well understood, it is thought to be a receptor phenomenon in which continued binding by a medication causes down-regulation of the receptor, which results in a decreased response to that medication. Stopping the medication for a short time for a drug holiday often restores the receptor's full functionality and thus re-establishes the medication's full activity.

RLS medications associated with tolerance include the dopamine agonists, opioids, and sedative hypnotics. When tolerance is suspected for any of these classes, it is often better to stop the medication for a few weeks instead of potentially worsening the problem by increasing the dose. When restarting the medication, using lower doses may be helpful to prevent the recurrence of tolerance.

Another strategy to prevent the recurrence of tolerance may be to take the medication on an intermittent basis, such as 3 to 4 days per week (often using the drug every other day). Since tolerance may occur from the constant bombardment of the drug's receptor, intermittent use may give the receptor frequent "mini" drug holidays, thus preventing tolerance from occurring. In fact, the intermittent medical use of opioids and benzodiazepines has not been shown to cause tolerance.

■ **Rotating Treatment**

The concept of rotating treatment shares the same mechanism as drug holidays. Both strategies are helpful for medications that may cause tolerance. When tolerance occurs with a dopamine agonist, changing to another may resolve the problem as cross-tolerance does not usually occur. However, some patients do develop tolerance to the replacement drug, at which point another one can be tried. It is not unusual for some patients to rotate two or three dopamine agonists every few months as they become less active. Many RLS patients have kept their treatment regimen potent for over a decade by rotating the agents.

Since cross-tolerance does occur with the benzodiazepines and opioids, this technique of rotating them would not work. However, some patients rotate the benzodiazepines or opioids with other drugs. This really is just simulating intermittent use of the drug as described for the mini drug holiday. The benzodiazepines can even be rotated with the opioids. They can be used on alternate days or 3 to 4 days in a row. While this rotation technique has never been formally studied, it may be considered for patients who have had problems with tolerance.

Referrals—When and to Whom?

When should you refer your RLS patient? The answer may differ depending upon the knowledge and comfort level of each physician. RLS is a disorder that should be diagnosed and treated by every primary care physician (PCP) similar to what one would do concerning other common diseases, such as asthma. A small percentage of all of these common diseases are referred to specialists when they are refractory to traditional therapy. As such, almost all patients with intermittent and daily RLS symptoms should be easily handled by their PCP.

Refractory patients may be somewhat more difficult. However, with the help of this chapter, PCPs may find that they can treat many of these cases. Treatment may require learning how to prescribe and maintain unfamiliar medications, but this task should be made easier by referring to the guidelines and detailed information in *Chapter 9*. As opioids are often required, prescribing their daily use may not be comfortable for some PCPs. Referrals to specialists should be made when, despite reading the guidelines and information available for treating such patients, the physician feels uncomfortable doing so.

As each physician treats more and more RLS patients, they may slowly feel more at ease treating the more complicated cases. Even with the benefit of this book, a physician must feel competent and comfortable in prescribing the recommended medications. When in doubt, it is better to refer the patient to a specialist and learn from the specialist. After seeing how the specialist treats these refractory patients, the PCP may gain sufficient knowledge and familiarity to treat these patients on their own.

To whom do you refer your patient? Unfortunately, no doctors are officially labeled as RLS specialists. However, there are many doctors who have spent years treating and doing research on RLS patients. Typically, neurologists, especially those who specialize in movement disorders, tend to have the necessary expertise for treating difficult RLS patients. They use all of the typical RLS medications, often in much higher doses, to treat Parkinson's disease and other neurologic disorders. Sleep-disorder specialists often see and treat numerous RLS patients, and most should have considerable expertise in this area, whatever their original speciality (internal medicine, psychiatry, neurology, or other). Many PCPs have taken an interest in RLS and have become proficient treating even the advanced cases.

However, the best way to ensure that the local neurologist, sleep specialist, or PCP with an interest in RLS is capable of treating these difficult, refractory cases is to talk directly with them. If they do acknowledge their expertise in RLS, you will be able to confirm their abilities by seeing how successfully they treat your patients.

REFERENCES

1. Hening WA. Restless legs syndrome: diagnosis and treatment. *Hosp Med*. 1997;33:54-56, 61-66, 68.
2. Silber MH. Restless legs syndrome. *Mayo Clin Proc*. 1997;72:261-264.
3. Chesson A Jr, Wise M, Davila D, et al. Practice parameters for the treatment of restless legs syndrome and periodic limb movement disorder. An American Academy of Sleep Medicine Report. Standards of Practice Committee of the American Academy of Sleep Medicine. *Sleep*. 1999;22:961-968.
4. Earley CJ. Clinical practice. Restless legs syndrome. *N Engl J Med*. 2003;348:2103-2109.
5. Silber MH, Ehrenberg BL, Allen RP, et al; Medical Advisory Board of the Restless Legs Syndrome Foundation. An algorithm for the management of restless legs syndrome. *Mayo Clin Proc*. 2004;79:916-922.
6. Lesage S, Hening WA. The restless legs syndrome and periodic limb movement disorder: a review of management. *Semin Neurol*. 2004;24:249-259.
7. Hening WA. Current guidelines and standards of practice for restless legs syndrome. *Am J Med*. 2007;120(1 suppl 1):s22-s27.
8. Aukerman MM, Aukerman D, Bayard M, Tudiver F, Thorp L, Bailey B. Exercise and restless legs syndrome: a randomized controlled trial. *J Am Board Fam Med*. 2006;19:487-493.
9. Sun ER, Chen CA, Ho G, Earley CJ, Allen RP. Iron and the restless legs syndrome. *Sleep*. 1998;21:371-377.
10. O'Keeffe ST, Gavin K, Lavan JN. Iron status and restless legs syndrome in the elderly. *Age Ageing*. 1994;23:200-203.
11. Hening W, Allen R, Earley C, Kushida C, Picchietti D, Silber M. The treatment of restless legs syndrome and periodic limb movement disorder. An American Academy of Sleep Medicine Review. *Sleep*. 1999;22:970-999.
12. Hening WA, Allen RP, Earley CJ, Picchietti DL, Silber MH; Restless legs Syndrome Task Force of the Standards of Practice Committee of the American Academy of Sleep Medicine. An update on the dopaminergic treatment of restless legs syndrome and periodic limb movement disorder. *Sleep*. 2004;27:560-583.

13. Trenkwalder C, Garcia-Borreguero D, Montagna P, et al; Therapy with Ropinirole; Efficacy and Tolerability in RLS 1 Study Group. Ropinirole in the treatment of restless legs syndrome: results from the TREAT RLS 1 study, a 12 week, randomised, placebo controlled study in 10 European countries. *J Neurol Neurosurg Psychiatry*. 2004;75:92-97.

14. Adler CH, Hauser RA, Sethi K, et al. Ropinirole for restless legs syndrome: a placebo-controlled crossover trial. *Neurology*. 2004;62:1405-1407.

15. Vignatelli L, Billiard M, Clarenbach P, et al. EFNS guidelines on management of restless legs syndrome and periodic limb movement disorder in sleep. *Eur J Neurol*. 2006;13:1049-1065.

16. Allen RP, Picchietti D, Hening WA, Trenkwalder C, Walters AS, Montplaisi J; Restless Legs Syndrome Diagnosis and Epidemiology workshop at the National Institutes of Health; International Restless Legs Syndrome Study Group. Restless legs syndrome: diagnostic criteria, special considerations, and epidemiology. A report from the restless legs syndrome diagnosis and epidemiology workshop at the National Institutes of Health. *Sleep Med*. 2003;4:101-119.

17. Hening W, Walters AS, Allen RP, Montplaisir J, Myers A, Ferini-Strambi L. Impact, diagnosis and treatment of restless legs syndrome (RLS) in a primary care population: the REST (RLS epidemiology, symptoms, and treatment) primary care study. *Sleep Med*. 2004;5:237-246.

18. Silber MH, Girish M, Izurieta R. Pramipexole in the management of restless legs syndrome: an extended study. *Sleep*. 2003;26(7):819-821.

19. Winkelman JW, Johnston L. Augmentation and tolerance with long-term pramipexole treatment of restless legs syndrome (RLS). *Sleep Med*. 2004;5(1):9-14.

10

11

Special Considerations

There are different groups of patients and situations that require special consideration. These include treating children and adolescents, the elderly, women who are pregnant or breastfeeding, surgical patients, and those with secondary restless legs syndrome (RLS) or periodic limb movement disorder (PLMD). Treatment plans have to be modified to avoid causing problems by fitting the special needs of these groups or situations.

Secondary RLS

Secondary RLS is defined as RLS that occurs due to another underlying medical condition. Typically, this includes three main conditions:
- Iron deficiency
- Renal failure
- Pregnancy.

As discussed in Chapter 3, *Who Gets RLS and How Does It Progress?*, several other neurologic and endocrine disorders may also be causes of secondary RLS. One of the goals for treating secondary RLS is to treat or resolve the primary condition. If that is not possible, the RLS is often treated similarly to idiopathic RLS, as long as the medications do not interfere with the underlying disorder.

■ Iron Deficiency With or Without Anemia

Iron deficiency as a cause of RLS was first noted by Nils Brage Norlander in 1953.[1] He found in an open-label study that large doses of intravenous iron provided 21 of 22 patients complete relief of their RLS for several months. O'Keeffe and colleagues next examined iron as therapy for RLS in an unblinded study in 1993 and found that oral iron therapy with ferrous sulfate 200 mg three times daily improved RLS symptoms.[2,3] They also discovered that the pretreatment level of serum ferritin determined whether patients responded to iron. Those with levels <18 mcg/L responded best, those whose levels were between 18 and 45 mcg/L responded but not as well as the lower ferritin group, and those with levels >45 mcg/L responded minimally. Another study performed by the Johns Hopkins group found that lower serum ferritin levels correlated with greater RLS severity, and all but one patient with severe RLS had serum ferritin levels <50 mcg/L.[4]

These studies have led us to check serum ferritin levels on RLS patients and treat them if the levels are <50 mcg/L. It should be noted that most laboratories report levels >10-20 mcg/L as normal. Additionally, many patients with iron deficiency do not have anemia[5] and the two studies discussed above did not find any significant correlation with serum iron levels and RLS severity.[2-4] Therefore, even when RLS patients present with no signs of iron deficiency (eg, anemia or low serum iron levels), a serum ferritin level should be assessed. Note that ferritin is an acute-phase reactant so it must be rechecked as it may be falsely elevated if the patient has any acute illness when drawn.

When serum ferritin levels are <50 mcg/L (even with a normal hemoglobin and serum iron level), oral iron supplementation is generally initiated with 325 mg ferrous sulfate, fumarate, or gluconate (65 mg of elemental iron) up to three times per day on an empty stomach with 100 to 200 mg of vitamin C, as tolerated. Many patients cannot tolerate oral iron, most often because of gastrointestinal side effects. However, for those who can tolerate oral iron, the goal is to raise serum ferritin levels >50 mcg/L. The serum ferritin level should be monitored periodically to avoid iron overload (ferritin levels >200 mcg/L). Iron repletion is to be avoided in patients with hemochromatosis, who are prone to accumulate toxic levels of iron. They may have a normal ferritin level, but their percent saturation will be notably elevated.

For those RLS patients with significant anemia that cannot be corrected with oral iron, intravenous iron dextran may be a reasonable choice as it has been demonstrated to improve symptoms markedly.[6,7] For other RLS patients, this therapy is still too experimental to be applied to those without resistant anemia.

■ Uremia

Secondary RLS in end-stage renal disease (ESRD) with uremia is common, with reported prevalence of up to 83%.[8,9] This can be a major clinical issue for ESRD patients who must sit for several hours a few times per week in their dialysis unit, despite the urge to move because of their secondary RLS. It has also been found that RLS may lower the quality of life and shorten survival in dialysis patients.[10] Clearly, it is important to treat RLS in these patients and it should not be overlooked.

As described in Chapter 9, *Medications and Other Medical Treatments*, there is ample evidence for improvement of the secondary RLS associated with ESRD through kidney transplantation.[11,12] However, this option is not available to most uremic patients and dialysis does not improve RLS symptoms. Therefore, these patients are treated somewhat similarly to those with idiopathic RLS, taking into consideration the interaction of their renal failure. In fact, most of the suggestions in the algorithm for managing daily RLS (see Chapter 10, *Approaching the Patient With RLS*), with some exceptions, may be followed for this group.

Nonpharmacologic Therapy

The steps of the nonpharmacologic therapies[13] outlined in Chapter 8, *Nonpharmacologic Management/Lifestyle Modifications*, and *Chapter 9* apply similarly to uremic patients. This group tends to be more anemic so iron and erythropoietin therapy may be helpful. One study showed temporary benefit (4 weeks) with high-dose IV iron dextran treatment[14] while other studies demonstrated improvement with erythropoietin.[15,16]

Dopaminergic Drugs

Just as with daily idiopathic RLS, dopaminergic drugs are considered the drugs of choice for uremic RLS.[8] L-dopa has been studied in uremic patients[17-20] and was found to be effective. However, other studies found that gabapentin[20] and ropinirole[21] were more effective than L-dopa for uremic patients. L-dopa may be used at the same doses as for primary RLS but similarly should be reserved for intermittent use (eg, just before dialysis a few times per week) to avoid the high risk of augmentation.

The dopamine agonists are among the most commonly used drugs for significant daily uremic RLS symptoms. Pergolide,[22] pramipexole,[23,24] and ropinirole[25] have been studied and found to be effective for uremic RLS. Ropinirole for uremic RLS can be used exactly as for primary RLS as it is metabolized in the liver and not excreted through the kidneys. Pergolide and pramipexole are both excreted through the kidneys so should be titrated more slowly and their maximum dose should be limited (0.75 mg for pramipexole). Just as for primary RLS, the ergot-derived dopamine agonists (pergolide, cabergoline, etc), due to their fibrotic side effects, should be considered only when the nonergot ones are not helpful.

Gabapentin

Two studies have demonstrated the benefits of gabapentin for uremic patients with RLS.[20,26] The drug was found to be more effective than L-dopa in this group and improved sleep, likely due to its sedative properties. Side effects were similar to those in treatment of primary RLS patients, although there is a report of two uremic patients developing myopathy.[27]

This drug is a reasonable alternative to the dopamine agonists. Due to its renal excretion, gabapentin should be given in a reduced dose of 100 to 300 mg after each dialysis.

Opioids

There are no studies on the use of opioids and uremic RLS. Although they may be as effective as for patients with primary RLS, they should be used with caution in ESRD patients since their active metabolites, which normally are excreted by the kidneys, will accumulate.

Benzodiazepines

The first and only study on the use of a benzodiazepine for uremic RLS was in a 1981 report on the benefits of clonazepam 0.5 mg in two split evening doses.[28] The authors found in this open trial that 14 of 15 uremic patients responded to 1 to 2 mg clonazepam daily, but that diazepam did not suppress the symptoms of RLS.

It is likely that the benefits of clonazepam are related to its improvement of insomnia. Similar to those with primary RLS, shorter-acting benzodiazepines or nonbenzodiazepines may be as effective and induce less daytime drowsiness.

11

■ Other Secondary RLS Conditions

As noted in *Chapter 3*, several other neurologic and endocrine disorders may also be causes of secondary RLS. For the most part, RLS that occurs in association with these conditions is treated similarly to primary RLS. However, for RLS associated with painful neuropathies, anticonvulsants, such as gabapentin or pregabalin,[29] may be more appropriate since they also treat the discomfort from the underlying neurologic disorder. In Parkinson's disease, the schedule of dopaminergic medications can be rearranged to facilitate treating RLS, but in most cases, it will be necessary to use the nondopaminergic medications (eg, anticonvulsants or opioids) to treat RLS.

As with uremia and iron deficiency, treating the underlying disorder may possibly benefit the secondary RLS symptoms. There is one report of a case of RLS that was associated with hyperparathyroidism with hypercalcemia that completely resolved after parathyroidectomy.[30] However, few reports reveal that treating other conditions improve secondary RLS.

Children

About 0.5% of children and 1% of adolescents suffer from RLS. Similar to the algorithm for treating adults, management should begin with nonpharmacologic therapy.[13] When possible, drugs that could potentially worsen RLS (sedating antihistamines, antinausea drugs, antidepressants, etc) should be avoided. Total caffeine restriction (including dietary items, such as chocolate) is suggested due to its effect on RLS and sleep.

Proper sleep hygiene may be very helpful for children. Iron therapy may also be beneficial and as noted with adults, serum ferritin levels should be evaluated. However, there are no guidelines for iron supplementation in children, so physicians should prescribe iron cautiously. The use of lower doses of iron, such as those available with multivitamins containing iron, may be a gentler alternative for treating younger children.

There are no guidelines for treating RLS in children with pharmacologic therapies, as several practice-standards articles have not found sufficient evidence to make any recommendations.[31-33] Children should only be treated with medication when RLS symptoms are severe enough to warrant therapy. Except for clonazepam, which is approved in children for treating seizures, all of the effective drugs are only approved in adults so their use is completely off label.

Due to their generally well-tolerated use in children with attention deficit/hyperactivity disorder (ADHD), clonidine and clonazepam have been used frequently in children with RLS. However, as newer drugs are now available, these older medications are prescribed much less often. L-dopa containing drugs have also been used with some success and are well tolerated,[34] but due to concerns of augmentation, they are used much less frequently in all age groups.

Currently, most specialists who treat children for RLS are using the dopamine agonists, ropinirole and pramipexole. A case study on the treatment of ADHD with ropinirole showed improvement of both ADHD and RLS symptoms in one child, and no adverse events were observed.[35] Studies of pramipexole for treating childhood RLS have yet to be published but one study found it to be well tolerated and effective for periodic limb movements (PLM) in six prepubescent children,[36] while similar results were found when treating two prepubescent children for night terrors and sleepwalking.[37] Both of these drugs should be used at their lowest possible dose (cutting the tablets in half may be reasonable) and increased very slowly.

11

Treating RLS in pregnant and breast-feeding women is often challenging due to the paucity of drugs that are safe in these groups. Care must be taken not to harm the fetus or child. Despite restrictions, there is adequate and safe therapy for these special populations.

■ **Pregnant Women**

As outlined in *Chapter 3*, RLS is common in pregnant women, especially in the second and third trimesters. RLS symptoms, which can be mild to severe, are superimposed upon the typical discomforts and problems that occur during pregnancy. At times, the disruption of sleep and added discomfort can be almost too much for some women to bear, even though symptoms usually remit within hours to days after delivery.[38]

Treatment begins with nonpharmacologic therapy similar to that for primary RLS. Serum ferritin levels are often decreased during pregnancy, but there are no studies showing benefit from treating with iron and one study revealed no benefit from iron therapy.[39] Another study that looked at iron and ferritin, folic acid, and vitamin B_{12} levels found that only low serum folic acid levels best correlated with RLS.[38] However, most women now take multivitamins that contain sufficient folic acid to avoid fetal neural tube defects. Nevertheless, physicians should check serum iron, ferritin, and folic acid levels in pregnant patients and treat them, if necessary, before starting drug therapy.

The use of medications should be reserved for very severe cases where the sleep disruption itself may cause prematurity and difficult delivery.[40] However, currently all of the guideline articles,[31,32] including the most current European Federation of Neurological Sciences (EFNS) article on the management of RLS,[33] state that there is insufficient evidence to make any treatment recommendations for RLS during pregnancy. Therefore, the following treatment suggestions are based on practical expert experience treating pregnant women with the few available reasonably safe drugs. When possible, drug use should be limited to the third trimester.

Medication should be chosen according to the Pregnancy Risk Categories outlined in **Table 11.1**. Since there are no safe Category A medications for RLS, the mildly risky Category B drugs are used.

TABLE 11.1 — FDA Risk Categories for RLS Drugs for Use in Pregnant Patients	
Risk Category	**Drug**
A	None
B	Cabergoline, pergolide (but limited data), zolpidem, methadone (low-dose), oxycodone (short-term use)
C	Pramipexole, ropinirole, rotigotine, levodopa, clonidine, zaleplon, eszopiclone, carbamazepine, gabapentin, propoxyphene, codeine, hydrocodone (all for short-term use), fentanyl, hydromorphone, morphine, demerol, levorphanol, tramadol
D	Alprazolam, clonazepam and most benzodiazepine sedatives; propoxyphene, codeine, hydrocodone, oxycodone (all for long-term use), methadone (higher doses)
X	Temazepam
Category A drugs have been tested and are considered completely safe in pregnancy; Categories B through D drugs represent degrees of danger and known teratogenicity, while Category X drugs are contraindicated in pregnancy.	

11

Pergolide is no longer available in the United States and cabergoline is very expensive. The other effective dopamine agonists are otherwise Category C drugs and should be avoided unless absolutely necessary.

Therefore, most RLS specialists prescribe opioids when necessary. Typically, low-dose methadone or oxycodone is preferred. Some experts prefer methadone since its use in high doses for pregnant addicts has already extensively been reported in the literature, including reasonable outcomes except for neonatal abstinence syndrome and prematurity.[41-43] Opioids must be discontinued late in the pregnancy, as they have been associated with neonatal withdrawal syndrome and respiratory depression.

■ Women Who Are Breast-feeding

Treating women who are breast-feeding their children presents difficulties, as many of the medications pass into the breast milk and may adversely affect the child. This includes gabapentin and other anticonvulsants, benzodiazepines, nonbenzodiazepine sleeping pills, most opioids (some have not been studied well enough for use in women who are breast-feeding), and tramadol. Methadone is considered reasonably safe in breast-feeding women due to its passing only minimally into breast milk. However, before prescribing methadone for severe RLS symptoms in this group, it might be more prudent to have them stop breast-feeding first.

Dopamine agonists cannot be used in nursing mothers as they decrease prolactin levels that in turn decrease breast milk production.

The Elderly

The elderly represent a very large group of RLS patients. According to the REST General Population Study, 64% of RLS sufferers were ≥50 years of age, with the peak prevalence increasing until age 79.[44]

The key issue with treating RLS in the elderly is their increased sensitivity and decreased ability to metabolize drugs. They often take multiple other medications, raising the risk for adverse drug interactions. As such, it is often wise to start with low doses (even ½ of the lowest-dose pills) and dose titration should be slower. The algorithm for the management of RLS[13] should be followed for this age group; however, opioids and hypnotics should be used more carefully as they may have increased adverse effects, such as falling.[45]

Another concern is that of secondary RLS since it has been found in >70% of those who have their RLS onset after age 65.[46] This group has been demonstrated to have faster progression of their disease, lower ferritin levels, and increased problems with neuropathy.[46,47] Serum ferritin levels <50 mcg/L were found in 58% of those with onset at >64 years of age compared with 22% of those with onset before age 50 years.[46] Therefore, new-onset RLS in the elderly should warrant a serum ferritin level test, and treatment with iron is suggested if it is <50 mcg/L.

11

Patients Undergoing Surgery or Outpatient Procedures

Surgical and outpatient procedures can be especially challenging for RLS patients and their physicians. Patients may have trouble staying still when at rest and PLM may cause problems with surgery or procedures. With proper care and knowledge, patients can be made comfortable throughout these procedures and problems are easily avoided.

■ Surgery
PLM is common in RLS patients and can occur during surgical procedures, even with spinal anesthesia.[48-52] This can make surgery very risky and thus

needs to be addressed. Usually, this can be resolved by the administration of an opioid (morphine) into the epidural or intrathecal space. Parenteral apomorphine is another alternative.

Medications that tend to exacerbate RLS are commonly used before and after surgery (especially antinausea drugs) and should be avoided as noted in *Chapter 8*. It is easy to choose a more RLS-friendly substitute that will not worsen the RLS.

For patients undergoing major surgical procedures, especially orthopedic ones, the chief concern is postoperative RLS symptoms caused by bed rest. Typically, this is not as much of a concern in the immediate postoperative period since opioids are used to treat the postsurgical pain. However, when the opioids are withdrawn, RLS symptoms quickly worsen, especially when patients remain somewhat immobilized. RLS medications need to be restarted as soon as patients can take oral medications. If they cannot take oral medications or if those drugs do not fully treat their RLS symptoms, parenteral opioids can be given. An alternative might be transdermal formulations of RLS medications.

Patients who develop RLS symptoms while under local anesthesia respond quickly to parenteral opioids or apomorphine. PLM may also improve with opioids but could do better with apomorphine.

■ Outpatient Procedures

Typically, MRI scans, CT scans, EEG/EMG tests, and many other outpatient procedures require patients to rest quietly for prolonged periods. Without proper treatment, this can be impossible for many RLS sufferers. However, pretreating with a dopamine agonist (1 to 3 hours before), L-dopa, or an opioid (30 to 60 minutes before) will usually prevent RLS symptoms or PLM from interrupting the procedure. As these procedures often provoke increased anxiety, a sedative may be added to one of the above drugs if necessary.

If RLS symptoms or PLM occur unexpectedly while the procedure is in progress, parenteral opioids or apomorphine should relieve them effectively and quickly.

Periodic Limb Movement Disorder

Over the past several years, whether or not to treat PLMD has become a very controversial issue. The sleep-specialty community is so divided that two pro and con debates among experts have been published on whether PLM should even be monitored in sleep studies[53,54] and whether PLM are associated with disturbed sleep and should be treated.[55,56]

The basis of this debate is that no study has demonstrated that PLM causes increased sleepiness or insomnia or that any benefit is derived from treating them. In fact, several studies have found that PLM may not be associated with insomnia, hypersomnia, waking up refreshed in the morning, the patient's perception of sleep quality, increased sleepiness on MSLT testing, or by subjective sleepiness scales.[57-59] However, recent studies have found that periodic limb movement in sleep (PLMS) transiently increases the heart rate by 7 to 10 beats/minute[60] and, more importantly, transiently increases blood pressure (an average of 11 mm diastolic, 22 mm systolic [and as much as 40 mm systolic])[61,62] which have been associated with vascular and cardiac damage.[63-65]

So how do we manage patients with PLM? This can be best done by dividing them into different categories. The first category is patients who come in because their bed partner complains about being kicked throughout the night and demands that something be done to resolve the situation. Typically, these are among the most motivated of people with PLM who

11

seek medical attention. If the person with PLM has no complaints of insomnia or hypersomnia, then RLS experts are divided on whether it is appropriate to treat them with medication (despite their demands for drug treatment). The simplest solution is for the couple to purchase twin-size beds and separate them by an inch at bedtime or invest in a king-size bed with a visco-elastic mattress (such as a TempurPedic). This should prevent the PLM kicks from disrupting the harmony of the relationship while allowing the couple to share a bed.

The second category of patients consists of those who complain that the PLM are vigorous and frequent enough to prevent their falling asleep or that they wake them up and then prevent their falling back to sleep. As these PLM occur while the patient is awake, there is no need to obtain a sleep study to verify the problem. These patients warrant a trial of drug treatment to see if their problem can be relieved pharmacologically.

The third category is comprised of patients who are very sleepy or who have insomnia and are not aware of their PLM other than from reports from their bed partner. Although the PLM may be responsible for their sleep problem, other conditions (eg, narcolepsy, sleep apnea, and REM behavior disorder) are also associated with PLM and need to be ruled out. Therefore, to warrant treatment these patients should have an overnight sleep study to determine that they do not have any other underlying sleep disorders and that the PLM are frequent enough and associated with arousals. There is also some controversy as to what frequency of PLM is abnormally high. Recent studies in older women (average age, 83 years) found that 52% of them had a PLM Index of >15/hour.[66] Therefore, it is not clear as to how many PLM per hour are necessary to warrant treatment. Most sleep specialists who do believe that PLM should be treated will usually consider treating patients when there are >40-50 PLM/hour associated with arousals (although this may vary considerably as there are no guidelines). If no other medical conditions or reasons can explain the patient's hypersomnia or insomnia, a trial of medication may be warranted to see if it helps the sleep-related complaints.

The last category is those patients who have a sleep study to rule out another condition, such as sleep apnea, and frequent PLM are reported. Similar to the patients above, if they have no other sleep disorder, yet have sleep-related complaints of hypersomnia or insomnia, a trial of drug therapy may be reasonable.

Before treating the patient for PLM pharmacologically, the physician should review the patient's current medications. Typically, antidepressants (especially the SSRIs and SNRIs) increase PLM,[67] and if medically appropriate, a change to bupropion (which does not worsen PLM) may be helpful. In addition, physicians should question patients further about RLS symptoms as this is a common association (>85% of RLS patients have PLM) that can be easily missed. If these patients need treatment for their RLS, those therapies will typically resolve their PLM at the same time.

For treating PLMD, the dopaminergic drugs (L-dopa, pergolide, pramipexole, and ropinirole) are considered effective to reduce the amount of PLM.[68] Most experts who treat RLS and PLMD consider ropinirole and pramipexole to be the most effective treatment for PLMD and one of the best-tolerated.

There is also evidence that gabapentin is effective for PLM.[69-71] Opioids help RLS symptoms but there are few studies on their benefits for PLM.[72,73]

Benzodiazepines have been used to treat PLMD, but although some studies show that they decrease PLM,[74-77] most other studies found that they do not decrease the amount of PLM but rather decrease the arousals caused by the PLM and improve sleep quality.[78-82] These studies were done using clonazepam, temazepam, and triazolam, and any of these medications would be a reasonable choice to treat a patient

11

with PLMD, especially if they complain about poor sleep quality or insomnia. However, similar to treating RLS, the shorter-acting benzodiazepines or nonbenzodiazepines may be preferred.

REFERENCES

1. Norlander NB. Therapy in restless legs. *Acta Med Scand.* 1953;145:453-457.
2. O'Keeffe ST, Noel J, Lavan JN. Restless legs syndrome in the elderly. *Postgrad Med J.* 1993;69:701-703.
3. O'Keeffe ST, Gavin K, Lavan JN. Iron status and restless legs syndrome in the elderly. *Age Ageing.* 1994 May;23(3):200-3.
4. Sun ER, Chen CA, Ho G, Earley CJ, Allen RP. Iron and the restless legs syndrome. *Sleep.* 1998;21:371-377.
5. Looker AC, Dallman PR, Carroll MD, Gunter EW, Johnson CL. Prevalence of iron deficiency in the United States. *JAMA.* 1997;277:973-976.
6. Earley CJ, Heckler D, Allen RP. The treatment of restless legs syndrome with intravenous iron dextran. *Sleep Med.* 2004;5:231-235.
7. Earley CJ, Heckler D, Allen RP. Repeated IV doses of iron provides effective supplemental treatment of restless legs syndrome. *Sleep Med.* 2005;6:301-305.
8. Kavanagh D, Siddiqui S, Geddes CC. Restless legs syndrome in patients on dialysis. *Am J Kidney Dis.* 2004;43:763-771.
9. Molnar MZ, Novak M, Mucsi I. Management of restless legs syndrome in patients on dialysis. *Drugs.* 2006;66:607-624.
10. Unruh ML, Levey AS, D'Ambrosio C, Fink NE, Powe NR, Meyer KB; Choices for Healthy Outcomes in Caring for End-Stage Renal Disease (CHOICE) Study. Restless legs symptoms among incident dialysis patients: association with lower quality of life and shorter survival. *Am J Kidney Dis.* 2004;43:900-909.
11. Yasuda T, Nishimura A, Katsuki Y, Tsuji Y. Restless legs syndrome treated successfully by kidney transplantation--a case report. *Clin Transpl.* 1986;:138.
12. Winkelmann J, Stautner A, Samtleben W, Trenkwalder C. Long-term course of restless legs syndrome in dialysis patients after kidney transplantation. *Mov Disord.* 2002;17:1072-1076.
13. Silber MH, Ehrenberg BL, Allen RP, et al; Medical Advisory Board of the Restless Legs Syndrome Foundation. An algorithm for the management of restless legs syndrome. *Mayo Clin Proc.* 2004;79:916-922.

14. Sloand JA, Shelly MA, Feigin A, Bernstein P, Monk RD. A double-blind, placebo-controlled trial of intravenous iron dextran therapy in patients with ESRD and restless legs syndrome. *Am J Kidney Dis*. 2004;43:663-670.

15. Harris DC, Chapman JR, Stewart JH, Lawrence S, Roger SD. Low dose erythropoietin in maintenance haemodialysis: improvement in quality of life and reduction in true cost of haemodialysis. *Aust N Z J Med*. 1991;21:693-700.

16. Benz RL, Pressman MR, Hovick ET, Peterson DD. A preliminary study of the effects of correction of anemia with recombinant human erythropoietin therapy on sleep, sleep disorders, and daytime sleepiness in hemodialysis patients (The SLEEPO study). *Am J Kidney Dis*. 1999;34:1089-1095.

17. Sandyk R, Bernick C, Lee SM, Stern LZ, Iacono RP, Bamford CR. L-dopa in uremic patients with the restless legs syndrome. *Int J Neurosci*. 1987;35:233-235.

18. Wetter TC, Trenkwalder C, Stiasny K, et al. Treatment of idiopathic and uremic restless legs syndrome with L-dopa—a double-blind cross-over study. *Wien Med Wochenschr*. 1995;145:525-527.

19. Trenkwalder C, Stiasny K, Pollmacher T, et al. L-dopa therapy of uremic and idiopathic restless legs syndrome: a double-blind, crossover trial. *Sleep*. 1995;18:681-688.

20. Micozkadioglu H, Ozdemir FN, Kut A, Sezer S, Saatci U, Haberal M. Gabapentin versus levodopa for the treatment of Restless Legs Syndrome in hemodialysis patients: an open-label study. *Ren Fail*. 2004;26:393-397.

21. Pellecchia MT, Vitale C, Sabatini M, et al. Ropinirole as a treatment of restless legs syndrome in patients on chronic hemodialysis: an open randomized crossover trial versus levodopa sustained release. *Clin Neuropharmacol*. 2004;27:178-181.

22. Pieta J, Millar T, Zacharias J, Fine A, Kryger M. Effect of pergolide on restless legs and leg movements in sleep in uremic patients. *Sleep*. 1998;21:617-622.

23. Miranda M, Fabres L, Kagi M, et al. Treatment of restless legs syndrome in uremic patients undergoing dialysis with pramipexole: preliminary results. *Rev Med Chil*. 2003;131:700-701.

24. Miranda M, Kagi M, Fabres L, et al. Pramipexole for the treatment of uremic restless legs in patients undergoing hemodialysis. *Neurology*. 2004;62:831-832.

25. Pellecchia MT, Vitale C, Sabatini M, et al. Ropinirole as a treatment of restless legs syndrome in patients on chronic hemodialysis: an open randomized crossover trial versus levodopa sustained release. *Clin Neuropharmacol*. 2004;27:178-181.

11

26. Thorp ML, Morris CD, Bagby SP. A crossover study of gabapentin in treatment of restless legs syndrome among hemodialysis patients. *Am J Kidney Dis*. 2001;38:104-108.

27. Lipson J, Lavoie S, Zimmerman D. Gabapentin-induced myopathy in 2 patients on short daily hemodialysis. *Am J Kidney Dis*. 2005;45:e100-e104.

28. Read DJ, Feest TG, Nassim MA. Clonazepam: effective treatment for restless legs syndrome in uraemia. *Br Med J* (Clin Res Ed). 1981;283:885-886.

29. Sommer M, Bachmann CG, Liebetanz KM, Schindehutte J, Tings T, Paulus W. Pregabalin in restless legs syndrome with and without neuropathic pain. *Acta Neurol Scand*. 2007;115:347-350.

30. Lim LL, Dinner D, Tham KW, Siraj E, Shields R Jr. Restless legs syndrome associated with primary hyperparathyroidism. *Sleep Med*. 2005;6:283-285.

31. Chesson AL Jr, Wise M, Davila D, et al. Practice parameters for the treatment of restless legs syndrome and periodic limb movement disorder. An American Academy of Sleep Medicine Report. Standards of Practice Committee of the American Academy of Sleep Medicine. *Sleep*. 1999;22:961-968.

32. Littner MR, Kushida C, Anderson WM, et al. Standards of Practice Committee of the American Academy of Sleep Medicine. Practice parameters for the dopaminergic treatment of restless legs syndrome and periodic limb movement disorder. *Sleep*. 2004;27:557-559.

33. Vignatelli L, Billiard M, Clarenbach P, et al. EFNS Task Force. EFNS guidelines on management of restless legs syndrome and periodic limb movement disorder in sleep. *Eur J Neurol*. 2006;13:1049-1065.

34. Walters AS, Mandelbaum DE, Lewin DS, Kugler S, England SJ, Miller M. Dopaminergic therapy in children with restless legs/periodic limb movements in sleep and ADHD. Dopaminergic Therapy Study Group. *Pediatr Neurol*. 2000;22:182-186.

35. Konofal E, Arnulf I, Lecendreux M, Mouren MC. Ropinirole in a child with attention-deficit hyperactivity disorder and restless legs syndrome. *Pediatr Neurol*. 2005;32:350-351.

36. Martinez S, Guilleminault C. Periodic leg movements in prepubertal children with sleep disturbance. *Dev Med Child Neurol*. 2004;46:765-770.

37. Guilleminault C, Palombini L, Pelayo R, Chervin RD. Sleep-walking and sleep terrors in prepubertal children: what triggers them? *Pediatrics*. 2003;111:e17-e25.

38. Lee KA, Zaffke ME, Baratte-Beebe K. Restless legs syndrome and sleep disturbance during pregnancy: the role of folate and iron. *J Womens Health Gend Based Med*. 2001;10:335-341.

39. Manconi M, Govoni V, De Vito A, et al. Restless legs syndrome and pregnancy. *Neurology*. 2004;63:1065-1069.

40. Manconi M, Ferini-Strambi L, Hening WA. Response to Clinical Corners case (Sleep Medicine 6/2: 83-4): Pregnancy associated with daytime sleepiness and nighttime restlessness. *Sleep Med*. 2005;6:477-478.

41. Wang EC. Methadone treatment during pregnancy. *J Obstet Gynecol Neonatal Nurs*. 1999;28:615-622.

42. McCarthy JJ, Leamon MH, Parr MS, Anania B. High-dose methadone maintenance in pregnancy: maternal and neonatal outcomes. *Am J Obstet Gynecol*. 2005;193:606-610.

43. Lejeune C, Simmat-Durand L, Gourarier L, Aubisson S; Groupe d'Etudes Grossesse et Addictions (GEGA). Prospective multicenter observational study of 260 infants born to 259 opiate-dependent mothers on methadone or high-dose buprenophine substitution. *Drug Alcohol Depend*. 2006;82:250-257.

44. Allen RP, Walters AS, Montplaisir J, et al. Restless legs syndrome prevalence and impact: REST general population study. *Arch Intern Med*. 2005;165:1286-1292.

45. Mendelson WB. The use of sedative/hypnotic medication and its correlation with falling down in the hospital. *Sleep*. 1996;19:698-701.

46. O'Keeffe ST. Secondary causes of restless legs syndrome in older people. *Age Ageing*. 2005;34:349-352.

47. Allen RP, Earley CJ. Defining the phenotype of the restless legs syndrome (RLS) using age-of-symptom-onset. *Sleep Med*. 2000;1:11-19.

48. Shin YK. Restless leg syndrome: unusual cause of agitation under anesthesia. *South Med J*. 1987;80:278-279.

49. Martinez LP, Koza M. Anesthesia-related periodic involuntary movement in an obstetrical patient for cesarean section under epidural anesthesia: a case report. *AANA J*. 1997;65:150-153.

50. Moorthy SS, Dierdorf SF. Restless legs during recovery from spinal anesthesia. *Anesth Analg*. 1990;70:337.

51. Watanabe S, Sakai K, Ono Y, Seino H, Naito H. Alternating periodic leg movement induced by spinal anesthesia in an elderly male. *Anesth Analg*. 1987;66:1031-1032.

52. Watanabe S, Ono A, Naito H. Periodic leg movements during either epidural or spinal anesthesia in an elderly man without sleep-related (nocturnal) myoclonus. *Sleep*. 1990;13:262-266.

53. Mahowald MW. Con: assessment of periodic leg movements is not an essential component of an overnight sleep study. *Am J Respir Crit Care Med*. 2001;164:1340-1341.

54. Walters AS. Pro: assessment of periodic leg movements is an essential component of an overnight sleep study. *Am J Respir Crit Care Med*. 2001;164:1339-1340.

55. Mahowald MW. Periodic limb movements are NOT associated with disturbed sleep. *J Clin Sleep Med*. 2007;3:15-17.

11

56. Hogl B. Periodic limb movements are associated with disturbed sleep. Pro. *J Clin Sleep Med.* 2007;3:12-14.

57. Mendelson WB. Are periodic leg movements associated with clinical sleep disturbance? *Sleep.* 1996;19:219-223.

58. Hilbert J, Mohsenin V. Can periodic limb movement disorder be diagnosed without polysomnography? A case-control study. *Sleep Med.* 2003;4:35-41.

59. Hornyak M, Riemann D, Voderholzer U. Do periodic leg movements influence patients' perception of sleep quality? *Sleep Med.* 2004;5:597-600.

60. Gosselin N, Lanfranchi P, Michaud M, et al. Age and gender effects on heart rate activation associated with periodic leg movements in patients with restless legs syndrome. *Clin Neurophysiol.* 2003;114:2188-2195.

61. Ali NJ, Davies RJ, Fleetham JA, Stradling JR. Periodic movements of the legs during sleep associated with rises in systemic blood pressure. *Sleep.* 1991;14:163-165.

62. Pennestri MH, Montplaisir J, Colombo R, Lavigne G, Lanfranchi PA. Nocturnal blood pressure changes in patients with restless legs syndrome. *Neurology.* 2007;68:1213-1218.

63. Frattola A, Parati G, Cuspidi C, Albini F, Mancia G. Prognostic value of 24-hour blood pressure variability. *J Hypertens.* 1993;11:1133-1137.

64. Zakopoulos NA, Tsivgoulis G, Barlas G, et al. Time rate of blood pressure variation is associated with increased common carotid artery intima-media thickness. *Hypertension.* 2005;45:505-512.

65. Roman MJ, Pickering TG, Schwartz JE, Pini R, Devereux RB. Relation of blood pressure variability to carotid atherosclerosis and carotid artery and left ventricular hypertrophy. *Arterioscler Thromb Vasc Biol.* 2001;21:1507-1511.

66. Claman DM, Redline S, Blackwell T, et al. Study of Osteoporotic Fratures Research Group. Prevalence and correlates of periodic limb movements in older women. *J Clin Sleep Med.* 2006;2:438-445.

67. Yang C, White DP, Winkelman JW. Antidepressants and periodic leg movements of sleep. *Biol Psychiatry.* 2005;58:510-514.

68. Littner MR, Kushida C, Anderson WM, et al. Standards of Practice Committee of the American Academy of Sleep Medicine. Practice parameters for the dopaminergic treatment of restless legs syndrome and periodic limb movement disorder. *Sleep.* 2004;27:557-559.

69. Happe S, Klosch G, Saletu B, Zeitlhofer J. Treatment of idiopathic restless legs syndrome (RLS) with gabapentin. *Neurology.* 2001;57:1717-1719.

70. Garcia-Borreguero D, Larrosa O, de la Llave Y, Verger K, Masramon X, Hernandez G. Treatment of restless legs syndrome with gabapentin: a double-blind, cross-over study. *Neurology*. 2002;59:1573-1579.

71. Happe S, Sauter C, Klosch G, Saletu B, Zeitlhofer J. Gabapentin versus ropinirole in the treatment of idiopathic restless legs syndrome. *Neuropsychobiology*. 2003;48:82-86.

72. Kaplan PW, Allen RP, Buchholz DW, Walters JK. A double-blind, placebo-controlled study of the treatment of periodic limb movements in sleep using carbidopa/levodopa and propoxyphene. *Sleep*. 1993;16:717-723.

73. Walters AS, Wagner ML, Hening WA, et al. Successful treatment of the idiopathic restless legs syndrome in a randomized double-blind trial of oxycodone versus placebo. *Sleep*. 1993;16:327-332.

74. Ohanna N, Peled R, Rubin AH, Zomer J, Lavie P. Periodic leg movements in sleep: effect of clonazepam treatment. *Neurology*. 1985;35:408-411.

75. Peled R, Lavie P. Double-blind evaluation of clonazepam on periodic leg movements in sleep. *J Neurol Neurosurg Psychiatry*. 1987;50:1679-1681.

76. Edinger JD, Fins AI, Sullivan RJ, Marsh GR, Dailey DS, Young M. Comparison of cognitive-behavioral therapy and clonazepam for treating periodic limb movement disorder. *Sleep*. 1996;19:442-444.

77. Horiguchi J, Inami Y, Sasaki A, Nishimatsu O, Sukegawa T. Periodic leg movements in sleep with restless legs syndrome: effect of clonazepam treatment. *Jpn J Psychiatry Neurol*. 1992;46:727-732.

78. Mitler MM, Browman CP, Menn SJ, Gujavarty K, Timms RM. Nocturnal myoclonus: treatment efficacy of clonazepam and temazepam. *Sleep*. 1986;9:385-392.

79. Bonnet MH, Arand DL. The use of triazolam in older patients with periodic leg movements, fragmented sleep, and daytime sleepiness. *J Gerontol*. 1990;45:M139-M144.

80. Doghramji K, Browman CP, Gaddy JR, Walsh JK. Triazolam diminishes daytime sleepiness and sleep fragmentation in patients with periodic leg movements in sleep. *J Clin Psychopharmacol*. 1991;11:284-290.

81. Bonnet MH, Arand DL. Chronic use of triazolam in patients with periodic leg movements, fragmented sleep and daytime sleepiness. *Aging* (Milano). 1991;3:313-324.

82. Saletu M, Anderer P, Saletu-Zyhlarz G, et al. Restless legs syndrome (RLS) and periodic limb movement disorder (PLMD): acute placebo-controlled sleep laboratory studies with clonazepam. *Eur Neuropsychopharmacol*. 2001;11:153-161.

12

RLS and Psychiatric Disorders

Introduction

As early as the 19th century, Wittmaack observed the co-occurrence of restless legs syndrome (RLS) with depression and anxiety, what he termed "anxietus tibiarum," and believed it to be a form of hysteria.[1] However, considered a rare neurologic disorder treated primarily by neurologists, psychiatrists rarely recognized or treated RLS. For example, most neurologists think that Ekbom's syndrome refers to RLS. However, psychiatrists are more familiar with Ekbom's syndrome as delusional parasitosis, a condition in which a person holds a belief that parasites have infested him or her.[2] This mix-up is due to the fact that Karl Ekbom, a Swedish neurologist, described both conditions separately, delusional parasitosis in 1937[3] and RLS in 1945,[4] and thus both conditions refer to him. Yet, this confusion also illustrates how the clinical entity of RLS lies in the boundary between psychiatry and neurology.

Recently, RLS has become increasingly important in the practice of psychiatry, as several studies have reported a high prevalence of psychiatric comorbidities among RLS sufferers, particularly depression and anxiety.[5] The purpose of this chapter is to provide an overview of the clinical aspects of managing RLS in this population, while highlighting emerging evidence for close association between RLS and psychiatric disorders.

Epidemiology of the Psychiatric Comorbidity of RLS

Epidemiologically, there are several striking similarities between RLS and mood disorders, especially depression. First, both RLS and major depression have similar prevalence in the community. Approximately 5% to 10% of the general population has RLS of varying severity,[6] and lifetime prevalence of major depressive disorder (MDD) in the community is between 5% to 10%.[7] Mean age at onset of both conditions is in the 30s with wide distribution.[6,8] Another interesting similarity is the female preponderance of 2 to 1 for both RLS and MDD.[7,9] Furthermore, both RLS and mood disorders have a strong genetic contribution to their etiology since multiple studies have confirmed family history as a strong risk factor.[10,11]

Therefore, it is not surprising that previous clinic-based studies reported a high prevalence of comorbidity between RLS and depression or anxiety disorders. Most of these studies relied on simple depression or anxiety rating scales with limited validity and did not have a control group, but their findings have been consistent.[5] Most notably, Winkelmann and colleagues, utilizing a structured psychiatric interview called the Munich-Composite International Diagnostic Interview for DSM-IV, assessed psychopathology among 130 RLS patients and compared the prevalence of MDD and panic disorder with 2265 residents who participated in community-based study.[12] The results from this study revealed an increased risk for having 12-month anxiety and depressive disorders with particularly strong associations for panic disorder, generalized anxiety disorder, and major depression (**Table 12.1**). This study focused on a clinical population, which likely had relatively severe RLS symptoms, and contrasted it to a select population sample of those with chronic somatic

TABLE 12.1 — Increased Risk of Psychiatric Disorders in RLS

Disorder	Increased Risk
Clinic-Based Sample in Germany[1]	
Panic disorder	OR=4.7 (95% CI=2.1-10.1)
Generalized anxiety disorder	OR=3.5 (95% CI=1.7-7.1)
Major depression	OR=2.6 (95% CI=1.5-4.4)
Community-Based Sample in Baltimore, MD[2]	
Panic disorder	OR*=12.9 (95% CI=3.6-46.0)
Major depressive disorder	OR*=4.7 (95% CI=1.6, 14.5)
Abbreviations: CI, confidence interval; OR, odds ratio.	
* These are adjusted odds ratio to account for possible confounds.	

[1]Winkelmann J, et al. *Sleep Med.* 2003;4:101-109; [2]Lee HB, et al. *J Neuropsychiatry Clin Neurosci.* 2007;48:167-169.

diseases. These results confirmed the high prevalence of depression and anxiety symptoms in RLS patients.

Several population-based studies have also reported increased rates of anxiety and depression in subjects with RLS.[5] Unlike clinic-based studies, population-based studies do not have a referral bias and have a comparison group drawn from the same population. Among the previous studies, the more recent RLS in Baltimore Epidemiologic Catchment Area (RiBECA) study provides strong evidence of the association between RLS and depression and/or anxiety disorder.[13] In this study, Lee and associates examined the association between RLS and DSM-IV MDD and panic disorder based on 1071 participants who completed the seven-item RLS Questionnaire and Diagnostic Interview Schedule. The study found strikingly high odds ratios in those endorsing RLS symptoms for both diagnosis of DSM-IV MDD and panic disorder in the past 12 months, suggesting a strong association between RLS and MDD and/or panic disorder (**Table 12.1**).

Potential Mechanism for Overlap Between RLS and Psychiatric Disorders

Recently, there has been much interest in a potential association between attention-deficit/hyperactivity disorder (ADHD) and RLS as well.[14] Several studies have reported that RLS and PLMS are common in children or adults with ADHD.[15,16] However, it is still unclear whether sleep disruption due to RLS rather than RLS itself is associated with ADHD-like symptoms of restlessness, overactivity, and inattention. One study compared ADHD symptoms in adults with RLS, normal controls, and controls with insomnia, and reported that ADHD symptoms are more common in patients with RLS than in patients with insomnia or normal controls.[17] However, diurnal symptoms of restlessness and inattentiveness of RLS could be mimicking ADHD symptoms on the rating scale without true attention deficits or hyperactivity.

Similarly, whether the close association between RLS and depressive symptoms is a by-product of symptomatic overlap remains an unresolved question. Out of nine symptoms listed for the diagnostic criteria for MDD in DSM-IV, RLS could trigger or exacerbate at least four of these depressive symptoms (**Table 12.2**).[5] On the other hand, according to the RiBECA study, MDD symptoms supposedly unrelated to RLS (**Table 12.2**) are just as common among those with comorbidity of RLS and MDD.[13] In other words, the association between RLS and MDD may be more than a superficial similarity due to the diagnostic overlap.

TABLE 12.2 — Overlapping and Distinctive Criteria for Depression With RLS

Depressive Symptoms That Overlap With RLS
- Insomnia or excessive sleepiness
- Decreased concentration, fatigue, or loss of energy
- Psychomotor retardation
- Dysphoric mood

Depressive Symptoms That Do Not Overlap With RLS
- Appetite loss
- Suicidal thoughts
- Low self-esteem
- Anhedonia
- Weight gain or loss

Alternatively, an underlying shared pathophysiologic mechanism between RLS and MDD might be responsible for the co-occurrence of RLS and MDD. Multiple studies have established the role of dopaminergic pathology in RLS.[18] Multiple studies also support a role for diminished dopaminergic neurotransmission in major depression in the following manner[19]:

1. Diminished dopamine release from presynaptic neurons or impaired signal transduction is implicated,

2. Animal models of depression show considerable responsiveness to dopamine neurotransmission,

3. Several studies have shown reduced concentration of dopamine metabolites in cerebrospinal fluid and in brain regions that mediate mood and motivation,

4. Neuroimaging studies have shown reduced dopamine transmission and compensatory upregulation of D_2 receptors.

In fact, bupropion, which has proven efficacy in the treatment of depression, acts, at least in part, via promoting dopaminergic function.[20] Several clinical trials recently reported a potential role for dopamine agonists, the first-line agent for RLS, for managing treatment-resistant depression or bipolar depression.[21]

The high prevalence of panic disorder in subjects with RLS is even more intriguing as little symptomatic overlap exists between the two conditions. Similarly, a high rate of comorbidity with panic disorder and MDD is observable in patients with Parkinson's disease (PD), a neurodegenerative disorder primarily involving central dopaminergic tracts.[22] Psychiatric comorbidities of PD can be attributable to direct dopaminergic deficits or interactions between dopaminergic deficits, as well as to the known variable deficits in norepinephrine and serotonin that occur in PD.[23] Little is known about the role of noradrenergic or serotonergic neurotransmission in the pathophysiology of RLS. Future investigations should examine the symptomatic and pathophysiologic overlap between RLS and MDD or panic disorder that frequently co-occur in the clinic and in the community.

Effect of Psychiatric Medications on RLS Symptoms

Since RLS and psychiatric disorders co-occur frequently, a clinician should give that fact careful consideration when choosing a medication for a psychiatric patient with comorbid RLS. Many psychiatric medications have the potential to affect RLS symptoms (see Chapter 8, *Nonpharmacologic Management/Lifestyle Modifications*). However, other than some case series or anecdotal reports, few studies have examined the direct effects of psychiatric medications on RLS symptoms, although several have examined the effect of these medications on the severity of periodic limb movements in sleep (PLMS). Since PLMS occur in at least 80% of RLS patients and correlate with RLS severity, effect on PLMS could be used to infer the effect of psychiatric medicine on RLS in general.

Predictably, all typical antipsychotics with dopamine receptor–blocking properties exacerbate PLMS. In fact, common antiemetics (eg, metoclopromide, promethazine, and prochlorperazine) also exacerbate RLS symptoms because of their dopamine receptor–blocking property. Newer atypical antipsychotics are less likely to exacerbate PLMS because of their lower binding affinity for the dopamine D_2 receptor, but two reports of initiation or exacerbation of RLS-like symptoms by risperidone and olanzapine exist.[25,26] Few data are available about effects of clozapine, quetiapine, and ziprasidone on RLS or PLMS. Aripiprazole, a partial dopamine agonist, theoretically might have a favorable effect on RLS symptoms, but no systematic study is available on this issue (see **Table 12.3** for a list of psychoactive drugs that may be more compatible with RLS).

Although various tricyclic antidepressants (TCAs) and selective serotonin reuptake inhibitors (SSRIs) have been suggested to exacerbate PLMS, it is unknown what specific mechanisms exacerbate PLMS.[5] Systematic studies have reported higher PLMS associated with TCAs, SSRIs, and venlafaxine.[27-29] Anecdotal reports of SSRIs and venlafaxine exacerbating RLS also exist.[30-32] In contrast, bupropion might alleviate RLS symptoms with its dopamine agonist mechanism[33] (**Table 12.3**). Trazodone also might have beneficial effect on RLS.[34] The effect of mirtazapine on RLS symptoms is unclear, as conflicting reports exist.[35]

Given the effects of these medications on RLS symptoms, it is important to screen for RLS symptoms before initiating antidepressant therapy. In fact, for a patient with severe RLS and mild depressive symptoms, it is reasonable to treat RLS first to see if improvement of sleep and energy lead to improvement of depressive symptoms. When treating depression in patients with severe RLS, clinicians should consider

12

TABLE 12.3 — Psychoactive Medications That Are More Compatible With RLS

Medication	Comments
Alternative for Neuroleptics	
Aripiprazole	Functions as a partial agonist at the dopamine D_2 receptor; some anecdotal claims have been made that it may help RLS, but studies are necessary to confirm this benefit
Alternatives for Antidepressants	
Bupropion	A weak dopamine reuptake inhibitor that may possibly help RLS symptoms,[1] but rarely worsens RLS[2]
Trazodone	This drug does not seem to affect RLS and may help sleep
Desipramine	Although TCAs tend to worsen RLS, the secondary amines, desipramine, protriptyline, and nortriptyline have less serotonergic effects and may be safer for RLS patients
Reboxetine	A selective noradrenergic thought to be neutral for RLS; although widely available, it is not approved in the United States
Nefazodone	This SNRI drug appears to have less serotonin effect than the others; not used very often due to its rare (1/300,000) side effect of liver failure

Abbreviations: SNRI, serotonin-norepinephrine reuptake inhibitor; TCA, tricyclic antidepressant.

[1]Kim SW, et al. *Clin Neuropharmacol.* 2005;28:298-301; [2]Picchietti D, et al. *Sleep.* 2005;28:891-898.

trying non-SSRI, or non-TCA antidepressants (eg, bupropion) initially. Yet, no comparative study of efficacy and safety involving bupropion and SSRIs in comorbidity of depression and RLS is available.

In the treatment of mood disorders, especially bipolar disorder, utilization of anticonvulsants (eg, valproic acid) to stabilize mood is common. In general, anticonvulsants associated with pain relief ameliorate RLS symptoms. Gabapentin and carbamazepine are second-line agents for the treatment of RLS.[37,38] Valproic acid might be also helpful in reducing RLS symptoms.[39] Several anecdotal reports of lithium exacerbating PLMS or RLS symptoms exist.[40,41]

Often, psychiatrists will prescribe benzodiazepines and hypnotics to treat insomnia related to psychiatric disorders, since these medications have not been shown to exacerbate PLMS. Among them, clonazepam is preferred over short-acting benzodiazepines because of its longer half-life. Studies that examined the effect of clonazepam on PLMS and RLS did not find consistent reduction in PLMS; patients instead reported a more restful sleep.[42] Commonly taken for sleep problems are antihistamines; however, diphenhydramine could exacerbate PLMS and RLS and should be avoided.[43]

12

Conclusion

RLS is a treatable, common disorder, closely associated with depression and anxiety in both clinics and community. Given the profound effect of various psychiatric medications on RLS symptoms, the psychiatrists treating psychiatric disorders in RLS patients should choose medications judiciously to avoid exacerbating RLS symptoms. Warranted are future systematic studies to guide clinicians in optimum treatment of psychiatric conditions, particularly depression and anxiety, in RLS patients.

REFERENCES

1. Wittmaack T. *Pathologie und Therapie der Sensibilitäts-Neurosen*. Leipzig: E Schäfer; 1861:459.

2. Enoch D, Ball H. *Ekbom's Syndrome (Delusional parasitosis) in Uncommon Psychiatric Syndromes*, 4th ed. London: Arnold; 2001:209-223.

3. Ekbom KA, Yorston G, Miesch M, Pleasance S, Rubbert S. The pre-senile delusion of infestation. *Hist Psychiatry*. 2003;14:229-256.

4. Ekbom KA. Restless legs: a clinical study. *Acta Med Scand Supplementum*. 1945;158:1-123.

5. Picchietti D, Winkelman JW. Restless legs syndrome, periodic limb movements in sleep, and depression. *Sleep*. 2005;28:891-898.

6. Allen RP, Picchietti D, Hening WA, et al. Restless legs syndrome: diagnostic criteria, special considerations, and epidemiology. A report from the restless legs syndrome diagnosis and epidemiology workshop at the National Institutes of Health. *Sleep Med*. 2003;4:101-109.

7. Robins LN, Helzer JE, Weissman MM, et al. Lifetime prevalence of specific psychiatric disorders in three sites. *Arch Gen Psychiatry*. 1984;41:949-958.

8. Burke KC, Burke JD Jr, Regier DA, Rae DS. Age at onset of selected mental disorders in five community populations. *Arch Gen Psychiatry*. 1990;47:511-518.

9. Berger K, Luedemann J, Trenkwalder C, John U, Kessler C. Sex and the risk of restless legs syndrome in the general population. *Arch Intern Med*. 2004;164:196-202.

10. Walters AS, Hickey K, Maltzman J, et al. A questionnaire study of 138 patients with restless legs syndrome: the 'Night-Walkers' survey. *Neurology*. 1996;46:92-95.

11. Winkelmann J, Muller-Myhsok B, Wittchen HU, et al. Complex segregation analysis of restless legs syndrome provides evidence for an autosomal dominant mode of inheritance in early age at onset families. *Ann Neurol*. 2002;52:297-302.

12. Winkelmann J, Prager M, Lieb R, et al. "Anxietas tibiarum". Depression and anxiety disorders in patients with restless legs syndrome. *J Neurol*. 2005;252:67-71.

13. Lee HB, Hening WA, Allen RP, et al. Restless legs syndrome is associated with DSM IV major depressive disorder and panic disorder in the community. *J Neuropsychiatry Clin Neurosci*. 2007;48:167-169.

14. Cortese S, Konofal E, Lecendreux M, et al. Restless legs syndrome and attention-deficit/hyperactivity disorder: a review of the literature. *Sleep*. 2005;28:1007-1013.

15. Chervin RD, Archbold KH, Dillon JE, et al. Associations between symptoms of inattention, hyperactivity, restless legs, and periodic leg movements. *Sleep*. 2002;25:213-218.

16. Picchietti DL, Underwood DJ, Farris WA, et al. Further studies on periodic limb movement disorder and restless legs syndrome in children with attention-deficit hyperactivity disorder. *Mov Disord*. 1999;14:1000-1007.

17. Wagner ML, Walters AS, Fisher BC. Symptoms of attention-deficit/hyperactivity disorder in adults with restless legs syndrome. *Sleep*. 2004;27:1499-1504.

18. Hening WA, Allen RP, Earley CJ, Picchietti DL, Silber MH; Restless Legs Syndrome Task Force of the Standards of Practice Committee of the American Academy of Sleep Medicine. An update on the dopaminergic treatment of restless legs syndrome and periodic limb movement disorder. *Sleep*. 2004;27:560-583.

19. Dunlop BW, Nemeroff CB. The role of dopamine in the pathophysiology of depression. *Arch Gen Psychiatry*. 2007;64:327-337.

20. Feighner JP, Meredith CH, Stern WC, Hendrickson G, Miller LL. A double-blind study of bupropion and placebo in depression. *Am J Psychiatry*. 1984;141:525-529.

21. Goldberg JF, Burdick KE, Endick CJ. Preliminary randomized, double-blind, placebo-controlled trial of pramipexole added to mood stabilizers for treatment-resistant bipolar depression. *Am J Psychiatry*. 2004;161:564-566.

22. Menza MA, Robertson-Hoffman DE, Bonapace AS. Parkinson's disease and anxiety: comorbidity with depression. *Biol Psychiatry*. 1993;34:465-470.

23. Cummings JL. Depression and Parkinson's disease: a review. *Am J Psychiatry*. 1992;149:443-454.

24. Allen RP. The resurrection of periodic limb movements (PLM): leg activity monitoring and the restless legs syndrome (RLS). *Sleep Med*. 2005;6:385-387.

25. Kraus T, Schuld A, Pollmacher T. Periodic leg movements in sleep and restless legs syndrome probably caused by olanzapine. *J Clin Psychopharmacol*. 1999;19:478-479.

26. Wetter TC, Brunner J, Bronisch T. Restless legs syndrome probably induced by risperidone treatment. *Pharmacopsychiatry*. 2002;35:109-111.

27. Garvey MJ, Tollefson GD. Occurrence of myoclonus in patients treated with cyclic antidepressants. *Arch Gen Psychiatry*. 1987;44:269-272.

28. Yang C, White DP, Winkelman JW. Antidepressants and periodic leg movements of sleep. *Biol Psychiatry*. 2005;58:510-514.

29. Winkelman JW, James L. Serotonergic antidepressants are associated with REM sleep without atonia. *Sleep*. 2004;27:317-321.

12

30. Bakshi R. Fluoxetine and restless legs syndrome. *J Neurol Sci.* 1996;142:151-152.

31. Sanz-Fuentenebro FJ, Huidobro A, Tejadas-Rivas A. Restless legs syndrome and paroxetine. *Acta Psychiatr Scand.* 1996;94:482-484.

32. Salin-Pascual RJ, Galicia-Polo L, Drucker-Colin R. Sleep changes after 4 consecutive days of venlafaxine administration in normal volunteers. *J Clin Psychiatry.* 1997;58:348-350.

33. Nofzinger EA, Fasiczka A, Berman S, Thase ME. Bupropion SR reduces periodic limb movements associated with arousals from sleep in depressed patients with periodic limb movement disorder. *J Clin Psychiatry.* 2000;61:858-862.

34. Saletu-Zyhlarz GM, Abu-Bakr MH, Anderer P, et al. Insomnia in depression: differences in objective and subjective sleep and awakening quality to normal controls and acute effects of trazodone. *Prog Neuropsychopharmacol Biol Psychiatry.* 2002;26:249-260.

35. Agargun MY, Kara H, Ozbek H, Tombul T, Ozer OA. Restless legs syndrome induced by mirtazapine. *J Clin Psychiatry.* 2002;63:1179.

36. Pae CU, Kim TS, Kim JJ, et al. Re-administration of mirtazapine could overcome previous mirtazapine- associated restless legs syndrome? *Psychiatry Clin Neurosci.* 2004;58:669-670.

37. Garcia-Borreguero D, Larrosa O, de la Llave Y, Verger K, Masramon X, Hernandez G. Treatment of restless legs syndrome with gabapentin: a double-blind, cross-over study. *Neurology.* 2002;59:1573-1579.

38. Telstad W, Sorensen O, Larsen S, Lillevold PE, Stensrud P, Nyberg-Hansen R. Treatment of the restless legs syndrome with carbamazepine: a double blind study. *Br Med J* (Clin Res Ed). 1984;288:444-446.

39. Eisensehr I, Ehrenberg BL, Rogge Solti S, Noachtar S. Treatment of idiopathic restless legs syndrome (RLS) with slow-release valproic acid compared with slow-release levodopa/benserazid. *J Neurol.* 2004;251:579-583.

40. Terao T, Terao M, Yoshimura R, Abe K. Restless legs syndrome induced by lithium. *Biol Psychiatry.* 1991;30:1167-1170.

41. Evidente VG, Caviness JN. Focal cortical transient preceding myoclonus during lithium and tricyclic antidepressant therapy. *Neurology.* 1999;52:211-213.

42. Saletu M, Anderer P, Saletu-Zyhlarz G, et al. Restless legs syndrome (RLS) and periodic limb movement disorder (PLMD): acute placebo-controlled sleep laboratory studies with clonazepam. *Eur Neuropsychopharmacol.* 2001;11:153-161.

43. Allen RP, Lesage S, Earley CJ. Anti-histamines and benzodiazepines exacerbate daytime restless legs syndrome symptoms. *Sleep.* 2005;28:A279.

13 Closing Remarks

RLS and Primary Care and Specialty Practices

It is our hope that this guide may assist both primary care physicians (PCPs) and specialists to manage diverse patients with restless legs syndrome (RLS). We expect that PCPs will become the main practitioners who treat RLS, or at least the majority of relatively uncomplicated cases. There are a number of benefits to treating these patients in primary care practice:

- RLS is a common condition that can be readily diagnosed in the clinic without extensive work-up
- RLS is responsive to therapy, so treating these patients can have a strong, positive impact on their lives.
- Treating RLS can be a gratifying experience for both the patients and physicians because of the speedy relief patients obtain from therapy.
- RLS patients are likely to remain with a physician who effectively treats their symptoms.

While we have provided information about patients who have difficulties with RLS therapy and the means of treating those patients, satisfactory management of the majority of RLS sufferers may require as little as a single medication taken for a period of years.

There are many specialties in which RLS can be a particular problem for the patients (**Table 13**.1). Optimal management of these patients will require that their RLS be addressed.

When diagnosis, severity, and management of RLS symptoms appear too complicated and require interven-

TABLE 13.1 — Specialities and Patient Groups Vulnerable to RLS

Obstetricians/gynecologists	Women who are pregnant have increased RLS; women, in general, have a 2-fold increased risk of RLS
Pediatricians	About 25% of familial RLS begins in the pediatric age range; children with ADHD are at increased risk for RLS
Oncologists/hematologists	Anemia and iron deficiency are related to RLS
Pulmonologists	Often involves sleep medicine, therefore, they must be aware of RLS
Internists/renal specialists	RLS is a major morbidity of dialysis; RLS associated with hypertension, cardiovascular disease
Psychiatrists	Psychoactive medications aggravate RLS; RLS associated with anxiety and depression
Endocrinologists	RLS is elevated in patients with diabetes and thyroid disorders
Neurologists	RLS is increased in Parkinson disease, multiple sclerosis, and neuropathy
Rheumatologists	RLS is increased in rheumatoid arthritis and other rheumatic conditions
Surgeons	RLS is increased by dopamine blocking and antihistaminergic medications used for sedation during procedures; RLS is increased in lung and heart transplants
Abbreviation: ADHD, attention deficit/hyperactivity disorder.	

tions with which the PCP (or non-RLS specialist) is uncomfortable, it is appropriate to refer patients to specialists who are more familiar with RLS. Neurologists (especially those trained in movement disorders) and sleep-medicine specialists (who may be neurologists, pulmonologists, or psychiatrists) are most familiar with RLS. Every sleep center is required to have expertise in diagnosing and managing RLS. Since not every neurologist or sleep-medicine specialist is truly an expert in RLS, it is useful to identify one who is comfortable in managing RLS. For children, pediatricians who specialize in sleep or neurology are most likely to be helpful.

Trends and Prospects

A major step in treatment of RLS was the approval of several medications, both in the United States and Europe. The two approved dopamine agonists, pramipexole and ropinirole, are effective and relatively safe medications for treating patients with this condition. They are the precursors to additional medications that may soon follow. Looking ahead, it seems likely that RLS pharmacotherapy will develop in two directions.

First, new medications may have a more extended duration of action. They either may have an increased half-life (extended-release versions of dopamine agonists) or be formulated for continuous release (rotigotine patch). Hopefully, such medications may avoid the difficulties with augmentation (see Chapter 9, *Medications and Other Medical Treatments*) that make daily treatment with levodopa highly problematic and even cause limitations for the immediate-release dopamine agonists now approved.

Second, there may the development of alternatives to the dopaminergic agents. Even though they remain the first-line treatment for RLS, dopaminergics may require supplementation with drugs from other classes, especially those already used for RLS in

13

past decades (eg, anticonvulsants, opioids, sedative hypnotics). A gabapentin prodrug may be approved in the next few years.

The availability of a wider range of approved medications will permit more flexible management of RLS. Together with various evidentiary reviews, these approvals will further legitimate the pharmacologic treatment of RLS. New evidentiary reviews—done by the Movement Disorder Society (together with the International RLS Study group and the World Association of Sleep Medicine) and the American Academy of Neurology—will supplement those done by the American Academy of Sleep Medicine[1,2] and the European Federation of Neurological Societies.[3]

Advances in RLS science are also likely, and they may have new and unexpected therapeutic implications. The unfolding of the relationship between brain iron deficiency and RLS[4] and the discovery of genetic variants predisposing one to RLS[5-7] provide just two lines of exploration that will likely expand our understanding of the biology of RLS. A PubMed search reveals that in a 6-month period (January through June, 2007), 105 articles associated with restless legs syndrome were published.

The opinions of those who regard RLS as a not-quite-real disorder that is being foisted upon a gullible public are likely to be made irrelevant (if not so already) by the developments in RLS clinical and basic science. The true clinical significance of RLS[8] is quickly gaining acceptance. We believe that RLS is likely to become categorized among the more important and common medical disorders. We certainly hope that our readers find that diagnosing and treating RLS becomes a routine and rewarding aspect of their practice.

REFERENCES

1. Chesson AL Jr, Wise M, Davila D, et al. Practice parameters for the treatment of restless legs syndrome and periodic limb movement disorder. An American Academy of Sleep Medicine Report. Standards of Practice Committee of the American Academy of Sleep Medicine. *Sleep.* 1999;22:961-968.
2. Littner MR, Kushida C, Anderson WM, et al.; Standards of Practice Committee of the American Academy of Sleep Medicine. Practice parameters for the dopaminergic treatment of restless legs syndrome and periodic limb movement disorder. *Sleep.* 2004;27:557-559.
3. Vignatelli L, Billiard M, Clarenbach P, et al.; EFNS Task Force. EFNS guidelines on management of restless legs syndrome and periodic limb movement disorder in sleep. *Eur J Neurol.* 2006;13:1049-1065.
4. Allen RP, Earley CJ. The role of iron in restless legs syndrome. *Mov Disord.* 2007. Epub ahead of print.
5. Winkelmann J, Schormair B, Lichtner P, et al. Genome-wide association study in restless legs syndrome identifies common variants in three genomic regions. *Nat Genet.* 2007;39(8):1000-1006.
6. Winkelmann J, Lichtener P, Schormair B, et al. Variants in the neuronal nitric oxide synthase (nNOS, NOS1) gene are associated with restless legs syndrome. *Mov Disord.* 2007. Lake Breaking Abstracts: 8.
7. Stefansson H, Rye DB, Hicks A, et al. A genetic risk factor for periodic limb movements in sleep. *N Engl J Med.* 2007;357(7): 639-647.
8. Hening WA, Allen RP, Chaudhuri KR, et al. The clinical significance of RLS. *Mov Disord.* 2007. In press.

13

Appendix A

The International Restless Legs Syndrome (IRLS) Study Group Rating Scale

The subject is asked, "In the past week..."*

1. Overall, how would you rate the RLS discomfort in your legs or arms?
   4—Very severe
   3—Severe
   2—Moderate
   1—Mild
   0—None

2. Overall, how would you rate the need to move around because of your RLS symptoms?
   4—Very severe
   3—Severe
   2—Moderate
   1—Mild
   0—None

3. Overall, how much relief of your RLS arm or leg discomfort did you get from moving around?
   4—No relief
   3—Mild relief
   2—Moderate relief
   1—Either complete or almost complete relief
   0—No RLS symptoms to be relieved

14

---

* It may be helpful to repeat the time frame with each question. One week is the time period most used for clinical trials; the original validation study used 2 weeks as the time period. Other time periods are possible, but if <1 week, question 7 may not work.

4. How severe was your sleep disturbance due to your RLS symptoms?
   4—Very severe
   3—Severe
   2—Moderate
   1—Mild
   0—None

5. How severe was your tiredness or sleepiness during the day due to your RLS symptoms?
   4—Very severe
   3—Severe
   2—Moderate
   1—Mild
   0—None

6. How severe was your RLS as a whole?
   4—Very severe
   3—Severe
   2—Moderate
   1—Mild
   0—None

7. How often did you experience RLS symptoms?
   4—Very often (6-7 days in 1 week)
   3—Often (4-5 days in 1 week)
   2—Sometimes (2-3 days in 1 week)
   1—Occasionally (1 day in 1 week)
   0—Never

8. When you had RLS symptoms, how severe were they on an average?
   4—Very severe (8 h or more per 24 h)
   3—Severe (3-8 h per 24 h)
   2—Moderate (1-3 h per 24 h)
   1—Mild (less than 1 h per 24 h)
   0—None

9. Overall, how severe was the impact of your RLS symptoms on your ability to carry out your daily affairs, for example, carrying out a satisfactory family, home, social, school or work life?

4—Very severe
3—Severe
2—Moderate
1—Mild
0—None

10. How severe was your mood disturbance due
to your RLS symptoms—for example, angry,
depressed, sad, anxious, or irritable?
4—Very severe
3—Severe
2—Moderate
1—Mild
0—None

Each question is scored from 0 for no problem or RLS or
symptoms to 4 for very severe. As a rough guide, the overall
score can be divided into different levels of severity:

0 .... No RLS
1-10 .... Mild RLS
11-20 .... Moderate RLS
21-30 .... Severe RLS
31-40 .... Very severe RLS

The scale can provide a single factor involving all of the
items summed.[1] It is also possible to divide the scale into a
symptom factor (sum of items 1, 2, 4, 6, 7, 8) and an impact
factor (sum of items 5, 9, 10).[2,3]

The IRLS is not a diagnostic instrument. It should only
be used after the diagnosis of RLS is confirmed. Since the
questions all refer to RLS, the patient must be aware of the
RLS symptoms and should be able to distinguish them from
other feelings or problems.

14

REFERENCES

1. Walters AS, LeBrocq C, Dhar A, et al; International Restless Legs Syndrome Study Group. Validation of the International Restless Legs Syndrome Study Group rating scale for restless legs syndrome. *Sleep Med.* 2003;4(2):121-132.

2. Allen RP, Kushida CA, Atkinson MJ; RLS QoL Consortium. Factor analysis of the International Restless Legs Syndrome Study Group's scale for restless legs severity. *Sleep Med.* 2003;4(2):133-135.

3. Abetz L, Arbuckle R, Allen RP, et al. The reliability, validity and responsiveness of the International Restless Legs Syndrome Study Group rating scale and subscales in a clinical-trial setting. *Sleep Med.* 2006;7(4):340-349.

Appendix B

Books, Web Information, Patient Organizations, and Resources for RLS

Books

Buchfuhrer MJ, Hening WA, Kushida CA. *Restless Legs Syndrome; Coping With Your Sleepless Nights*. New York: Demos Medical Publishing; 2006.

   Written for patients, this book covers the full spectrum of RLS topics including diagnosis, clinical features, pathogenesis, history, treatment (both drug and nondrug), relationships, disability, and children. With its many useful resources and detailed descriptions on how to treat many difficult RLS situations, it is also suitable reading for primary care physicians.

Chaudhuri KR, Odin P, Olanow CW. *Restless Legs Syndrome*. New York: Taylor & Francis; 2004.

   This is the first professional-level book written on RLS. Written by a panel of experts, *Restless Legs Syndrome* focuses on the diagnosis and management of RLS. The authors discuss the epidemiology of RLS, pathophysiology, clinical associations, and clinical features. They explore how to diagnose the many different types of people who present with this disorder. It includes discussions of the wide range of treatment options available in order to give clinicians the information they need to formulate appropriate pharmacologic or nonpharmacologic thera peutic regimens.

Gunzel J. *Restless Legs Syndrome: The RLS Rebel's Survival Guide. Tucson, AZ:* Wheatmark, Inc; 2006.

   This book describes the RLS Rebel Program, an outline that helps RLSers (people with RLS) organize their fight against RLS and achieve maximum results from any

15

combination of RLS treatments. When treatments include use of prescription drugs, the RLS Rebel Program becomes the ultimate complementary-medicine approach to RLS. The book includes six steps for reducing aggravating variables, suggestions for developing and using a "bag of tricks" approach, tips for better communication with medical professionals, advice to supporters of RLSers, suggestions for using the RLS Rebel Program in children, and information about dealing with RLS on long trips and in other special situations.

Ondo WG. *Restless Leg Syndrome (Neurological Disease and Therapy)*. New York: Informa Healthcare/Taylor & Francis; 2006.

This book, edited by William Ondo, is an authoritative and comprehensive guide on RLS. It examines the pathogenesis, diagnosis, and treatment the disorder. Ranging from basic science to therapeutics, this book analyzes the many new and emerging medications impacting the management of this disorder and strives to address the explosion of research in the field.

Wilson VN, Walters AS, eds. *Sleep Thief, Restless Legs Syndrome*. Orange Park, FL: Galaxy Books Inc; 1996.

This is the first book published on RLS. Written by one of the founders of the RLS Foundation, it contains both a layperson's perspective and professional essays from a variety of medical experts.

Yoakum R. *Restless Legs Syndrome: Relief and Hope for Sleepless Victims of a Hidden Epidemic*. New York: Simon & Schuster; 2006.

This book details the reality of RLS and its problems, as well as reviewing coping, therapy, and the science of RLS. It brings alive the real suffering of the patient with severe RLS and includes a multitude of individual testimonies. The author is a former member of the Board of Directors of the RLS Foundation and author of the historical article on RLS published in *Modern Maturity* in 1994. He prepared this volume in consultation with a variety of RLS experts, including members of the RLSF Medical Advisory Board.

The Official Patient's Sourcebook on Restless Leg Syndrome.
San Diego, CA: Icon Health Publications; 2002.

This volume draws from public, academic, government, and peer-reviewed research; provides guidance on how to obtain free-of-charge, primary research results as well as more detailed information via the Internet. Ebook and electronic versions of this sourcebook are fully interactive with each of the Internet sites mentioned.

Web-Based Information

American Academy of Sleep Medicine (AASM)
www.aasmnet.org

The American Academy of Sleep Medicine is the premier organization devoted to the advancement of sleep medicine and sleep-related research. It also serves as the key resource for public and professional education on sleep disorders. The AASM's educational website is at www. sleepeducation.com (which also includes patient information and on-line forums), and individuals with sleep problems can locate the sleep center nearest to them at www.sleepcenters.org.

Bandolier Website
www.jr2.ox.ac.uk/bandolier

Bandolier is a publishing company that has print and Internet versions of medical articles. By typing RLS in its search box, you will find reviews of many articles on RLS.

Johns Hopkins Center for RLS
www.neuro.jhmi.edu/rls

This website has educational and research information on RLS. Johns Hopkins is the most active center doing research on the role of dopamine and iron in RLS.

15

National Institutes of Health (NIH)
www.nih.gov

The NIH, a part of the US Department of Health and Human Services, is the primary federal agency conducting and supporting medical research. Many other organizations make up the NIH, covering different health specialties. Two of these offer valuable information on RLS:

National Institute of Neurological Disorders and Stroke
(NINDS) www.ninds.nih.gov

The NINDS website contains a wealth of information on neurologic disorders. The site contains a Restless Legs Syndrome Information Page (*www.ninds.nih.gov/ disorders/restless_legs/restless_legs.htm#What_is*) and a Restless Legs Syndrome Fact Sheet Page (*www.ninds.nih. gov/disorders/restless_legs/vdetail_restless_legs.htm*).

The National Heart, Lung, and Blood Institute (NHLBI)
www.nhlbi.nih.gov/index.htm

The NHLBI has a sleep section (*www.nhlbi.nih.gov/health/ public/sleep/rls.htm*) where you can download or order a free 4-page pamphlet Fact Sheet on RLS. They also have another Web page (*www.nhlbi.nih.gov/health/prof/sleep/ rls_gde.htm*) where you can download or order a free hard copy of this 16-page document called *Restless Legs Syndrome: Detection and Management in Primary Care*.

Patient Organizations and Web Resources

RLS Foundation
www.rls.org

The RLS Foundation is the international nonprofit RLS organization based in Rochester, Minnesota, that has advocated for and helped RLS patients since its inception in 1992. Their website contains information for patients on every aspect of RLS, including a list of doctors who treat RLS. Brochures can be obtained on many RLS topics and they publish a quarterly newsletter, *NightWalkers.* They also supply a medical-alert card that details the drugs that patients should avoid.

In addition to supporting patients, the RLS Foundation helps doctors with research grants for RLS, provides a quarterly scientific bulletin, brochures, and other information to aid in the treatment and understanding of this disorder. Physicians can join a list of medical providers who treat RLS, which may increase their access to RLS patients.

RLS Foundation Pamphlets and Videos
Living with RLS
Surgery and RLS
Depression and RLS
Pregnancy and RLS
Children and RLS
Medical Bulletin (reviews RLS treatment)
RLS Scientific Bulletin (reviews RLS research and new treatments)
RLS: Detection & Management in Primary Care (NIH document)
Understanding & Diagnosing RLS (video)

The Foundation hosts a forum and chat room where RLS patients can discuss their experiences with others. In addition, it sponsors support groups all over the world, trains support group leaders, and gives financial and educational help.

Currently there are over 100 support groups in the United States and Canada and several international support groups that work in cooperation with the RLS Foundation. These support groups can be invaluable for patients in many ways. As noted, they help decrease the isolation that RLS sufferers feel and validate that they do indeed have a real disease that is no laughing matter. They can learn about which local doctors are adept at treating RLS, non-pharmacologic therapies (eg, stretches or exercises) that may be beneficial, new drug treatments that are available, and other educational issues. Support groups can also be a forum for patients to share their bad times and successes battling their "tortured limbs." Every patient who has significant RLS is encouraged to join a local support group. If there is not one in their area, encourage the patient to start one (the RLS Foundation will help in doing so).

15

For patients who are too far from one of the support groups or who do not have the mobility to travel, there are internet support groups and chat/forums that can fulfill this need. Following is a list of these internet sites.

Brain Talk Communities
http://brain.hastypastry.net/forums

Cyberspace RLS Support Group
http://health.groups.yahoo.com/group/rlssupport/

HealthBoard.com
www.healthboards.com

RLS-PLMD at Yahoo Groups
http://health.groups.yahoo.com/group/RLS_PLMD

National Sleep Foundation
www.sleepfoundation.org
> The National Sleep Foundation has a wealth of sleep information and an RLS article reviewed by Richard Allen, PhD and Merrill M. Mitler, PhD.

Talk About Sleep
www.talkaboutsleep.com
> This site covers many sleep topics, including RLS. It also has chat rooms and message boards on RLS/PLMD topics.

The RLS Rebel Website
www.rlsrebel.com
> This site is written by Jill Gunzel, aka the "RLS Rebel," and is a must read for all people with RLS. Jill has suffered from RLS for over 40 years and has a innovative approach for treating RLS. Included are many novel tricks to combat RLS symptoms.

The Southern California RLS Support Group
www.rlshelp.org
> This site contains detailed information about the drugs used for RLS and has pages of letters from people all over the world with medical replies from an author of this book, Mark J. Buchfuhrer, MD. Patients can download free medical-alert cards from this site.

INDEX

NOTE: RLS stands for Restless Legs Syndrome.
Page numbers in *italics* refer to figures.
Page numbers followed by a t indicate tables.

16

16

16

16

276

16

16

16

16

16

16

16

16

16

16

16

16

16

16